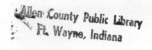
Photo Credits

Front cover: upper left, Johnson Products; upper right, Susan Wood Gearhart; lower left, Peter Estersohn; lower right, Deirdre Somer.
Back cover: upper left, Gabrielle Gearhart; upper right, Pivot Point; lower left, Renzo Renzi; lower right, Pivot Point.

ABOUT THE AUTHOR

Susan Gearhart is a professional model, dancer, and freelance writer and editor. She graduated from City University of New York and attended Hiram College, Juilliard School of Music, and the Preibar Academy in Berlin, Germany. She has worked as a professional model since her teens and has covered the field from artist's model to television to runway work. She has modeled for a wide variety of products, from cosmetics to bathing suits, and has made a career of freelance, agency work, part-time, and full-time jobs.

PREFACE

In America, the words "model" or "modeling" usually conjure up visions of extremely tall, young, thin blond women with blue eyes, long legs, and toothy smiles. The truth is that the world of modeling encompasses every color, size, shape, sex, and age group—and even every kind of animal. If it moves, it attracts the human's attention, and that is the idea behind every ad.

Appeal to the viewer sells the product, and ad agencies must promote the gimmick that most often catches the public's eye. One popular eye-catcher is the winsome blond whose look convinces you that either you could look like her or you could attract her if you buy the particular item she is appearing with. This model, with all the right appeal, can potentially make an income of $100,000 to $1,000,000 a year. The tremendous pay scale at the top in the modeling industry is certainly one of its greatest attractions.

Though the model described above is almost *the* exclusive big moneymaker in modeling, there are also a handful of stunning brunettes who have enough appeal to make it to the top.

There are also thousands of other models who work in every capacity from television commercials to retail store promotions, are paid very well, and enjoy their work immensely. This book describes the entire scope of the modeling profession to give you an idea of where you might fit in, or make your own new job slot, in modeling.

ACKNOWLEDGMENTS

My gratitude and appreciation are extended to the following for their kindness, help, and time: Bernie Bennet and Donna Templeton of Kay Model's agency; Hillary Cummings, model; Sarah Edwards, model; Magi English, researcher, London, England; Pieter Estersohn, photographer; Zoe Faircloth of Papillon School of Modeling, Asheboro, N.C.; Richard Feenstra, model; Gabrielle Marguerite Gearhart, model; Joe Hunter of Ford Men, Ford Models, Inc.; Miss Mancini of John Robert Powers; James Mischka, model; Mary Nolan; Chazz Norwood, model; Renzo Renzi, photographer; Deirdre Somers, international model; Carey Stokes, model for Ford Men, Ford Models, Inc.; *Teen Magazine;* and Barbara W. Donner, editor, National Textbook Company.

FOREWORD

This book is a "must read" for every potential and professional model.

Ms. Gearhart has a knack for getting to the most important, yet usually overlooked, advice that any of us within the industry could offer.

She gives the reader a balanced assessment of a potentially unbalanced business. Her emphasis on hard work and commitment to realistic goals is a very needed message in today's fashion market. An industry that is built on such amorphous ideas as beauty, style, imagination and impulse may be glamorous to the consumer; but it takes a special person to keep their feet on the ground—while portraying an *image* of one with their head in the clouds. Ms. Gearhart also reminds us of a realistic evaluation of ourselves. After all, "popularity must not be confused with possible modeling qualifications."

The major idea you, the reader, will remember—long after you have read this book—is a sense of reality within the business of fantasy. The fashion model is an actor in every sense. You will be portraying a character to your public, whether that character be sultry, classic, sporty or comic.

Ms. Gearhart reminds us that in fashion—*image* is our business. As a business it must be approached with the same realistic goals we would set in any other career—but, we never forget that fashion is also to be enjoyed.

Shirley Hamilton
Shirley Hamilton Inc., Talent Representation

INTRODUCTION

The very first models ever used were perhaps completely unaware that they were being used as the subjects of some primitive cave rendering. As later people became more sophisticated with their methods of depicting what they saw in the world around them, they employed human models to "sit" for them, in order to copy likenesses more readily. After awhile, it became more prestigious to be the model, as the person was often immortalized by the masters, in oil paintings, charcoal drawings, and sculptures. Museums house the likenesses of thousands of personages who would never have been so wonderfully remembered had they not been the subjects of artists' creations.

Modeling today has become a wide-spread profession encompassing every corner of the artistic to the commercial world. Models are paid wages for their work on a very individualized scale. Depending on the demand for the notoriety that each has developed, the payment could run from a minimal hourly wage to an annual income of hundreds of thousands of dollars. There are literally endless possibilities for modeling jobs, and if you desire work in this field, there is a niche that will suit you. The trick is merely for you to take honest stock of all of your assets and drawbacks and evaluate which is the niche for you.

DEDICATION

To Marguerite S. and Wm. Barker Wood,
Gabrielle, Jennifer, and Ted

CONTENTS

Artistic modeling. Illustrators modeling. Promotional modeling. Seventh Avenue modeling. Photographic modeling. Fashion show and runway modeling. Television modeling. Video modeling.

General attitude and dress. Physical qualifications for high fashion. Specific qualifications for all models. The specific qualifications for the male model. Specific qualifications for child models. Specific qualifications for the television model.

How do you know if you have what it takes? The beauty contest. Heading straight for the big agencies. Breaking into television modeling.

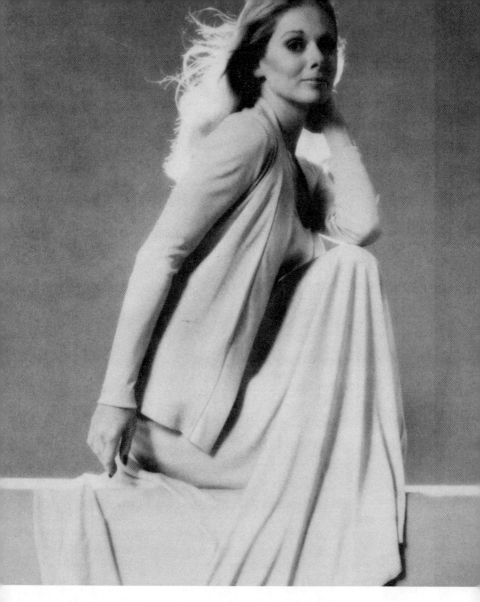

Model Sandie Wolsfeld does modeling for print media, commercials, and films.
Photo: Chic Inc., by Gremmler

CHAPTER 1

WHO ARE PROFESSIONAL MODELS?

There is a large field open to anyone who is interested in modeling. The different areas include artistic modeling, illustrators modeling, promotional modeling, Seventh Avenue modeling, photographic modeling, fashion show and runway modeling, television modeling, and video modeling.

ARTISTIC MODELING

If the idea of posing for long periods of time and having a real appreciation of an artist's temperament are within your grasp, you could probably find work sitting for life classes at your local art school, high school, photographic school, college, or university. You could also be privately employed by artists and sculptors for work in their studios. There are no regulations as to figure, size, shape, age, race, or often experience. The artist may need a particular type for the work to be created, but literally anyone could be hired to model for a given piece.

As an artist's model, you would be expected to be available to the classes or the individual artist until the work is completed. You would also have to be able to remain absolutely motionless for extended periods of time.

1

This is critical for the artist, so if you doubt your physical abilities, serious consideration should force you to look elsewhere for work.

There seems to be a lack of child models in art schools—and for good reason. They do not sit still long enough. But this does not disqualify them for the fashion drawing classes, as that is a critical part of the industry.

Most models are between the ages of eighteen and eighty and could quite reasonably make a full-time career of the work available. There are many art schools, art classes in museums, and private artists who work almost exclusively with experienced models. So the demand is greater than you might expect.

In New York, there are many institutes for fashion design instruction, and therefore many models are needed. Anyone could work in the many facets of the art classes, but fashion classes would have specific requirements.

Life classes, drawing classes, painting classes, and sculpture classes all require the real model who could be anyone on the street. Fashion classes require a fashion figure and the wardrobe (which you must supply) currently in vogue. There are also illustration classes where you would be expected to provide costumes. The model for these classes obviously does not have to have the figure of a high fashion model, but should be reasonably trim and attractive.

The pay scale in the New York area seems to be around six dollars per hour and if you are in demand, you could work as much as six hours a day, every day. The best approach to this type of work is to make an appointment with any of the many art schools listed in your phone book. They are generally helpful, even if they themselves do not currently need more models, and will tell you of other institutions and individuals who might. You could also put your credentials on the bulletin boards of places frequented by art students or professional artists—art stores, art institution bookstores, etc.

Some of the ways to be a popular artist's model are to remember that this is a business and to be prompt, fresh and clean, polite, and serious about your work. If you want to remain employed, professionalism is first.

Word of mouth is always your best advertisement. Visit art shows where you can actually meet the painters, attend an art class (students are very often chosen from the class to pose for each other) or simply call every art school, high school, and university in your area for information.

ILLUSTRATORS MODELING

This area of modeling incorporates the live model into a fantasy layout or some sort of not quite true-to-life picture. Illustrators are artists who use the model as the basis of the picture but deviate in ways that are required by the ad itself, or by embellishing or reducing the real characteristics of the model. Some works done by illustrators are so incredibly unlike their subjects that you would never guess who the model was.

In fashion work the rendering is usually far more ethereal, more animalistic, or more sensational than any human being could possibly look. Robert Petty was famous for creating the gorgeous women that took people's imaginations in the 1940s; Erte was a famous illustrator of the 1930s. Today, many fashion illustrators are kept busy with the demands of advertising agencies. Few people recognize who the artist is, and they take for granted many talented portrayals.

If you are hired to model for a fashion illustrator, you will be doing similar work to that of posing for a painter or sculptor. The main difference is that the illustrator is paid a very high price for renditions for an advertising agency, and thus your pay scale could be extremely high.

Another plus here is that this has nothing to do with your own body's perfection; you could work for an illustrator even if it's only your flaming red hair that has attracted attention to you as a subject. Often a fashion illustrator is hired to depict one particular angle of a garment, a certain color, or even a mood, and the illustration that results has little to do with the actual model. This must not be taken personally. You are merely the framework upon which the artist builds an idea. A model is able to move into positions that a dummy could never assume, and that is the bottom line in some of your modeling work.

The pay can range from $20 to $150 an hour for a few hours of playing movable dummy and the variety of the work is fun if you work with several illustrators.

PROMOTIONAL MODELING

The next large group of live models are those who do promotional work. These people are hired by agencies or directly by the company whose product they are expected to wear or demonstrate. These models could range in age from eighteen (though sometimes toys and various food products are shown by children) to elderly. The hourly wage is set by the employer, and it could vary from around ten dollars in the smaller cities to several hundred per hour in major cities, depending on the actual product and the prestige of the promotion. In some cities there are constant promotions that call for live models who are able to explain or "sell" a product. So verbal skills and a pleasant voice are a requirement for many promotional spots. The Colosseum at Columbus Circle in New York City has shows year-round that involve hundreds of live models at each show. These are a way for many students, actors, dancers, full-time professional models, and men and women who simply enjoy the work to make excellent money. The way to locate these particular positions is by reading trade papers or by keeping in touch with the annual promoters after having made contact during one of the trade shows. Modeling agencies also supply models for some of the bigger shows like the Automobile and Boat Shows. These jobs can be fun; they can also be downright exhausting, as you are constantly in front of the public and you must look pleasant for very long hours. The daily schedule is sometimes eight hours long, and you are usually expected to be on your feet and moving from one prospective customer to the next. The bigger shows run for a week at a time, so there is a sizable income to be made if you are working frequently. Every time you model for shows as large as these, you will be able to make many contacts for future modeling work.

In-store promotions are another area that uses many models, both men and women. The hours are usually only the busiest ones of the day, so that you will be able to introduce the new product to as many people as possible during the promotion. Most models hired for this type of work have to have verbal skills. They are responsible for explaining why the potential customer should use the product, and they must have a varied talk so that if a customer returns the model doesn't seem to have a totally "canned" speech. This type of modeling is rapidly becoming one of the largest and best-paid areas of the industry. The hours are guaranteed to be fairly extended as you demonstrate varied products in endless department stores.

In the smaller cities as well as the larger ones, promotional models are evident. The model is hired by the company whose product he or she will demonstrate. The contact from the company may be direct or may come through modeling agencies. If you think that you might like in-store promotional work, ask a model doing such work how he or she became employed. In New York, there are so many of these jobs available that certain agencies handle these models exclusively. In smaller cities, you could contact the personnel department in the store itself or ask the promoter directly. Modeling schools often put on these shows, and you might want to call them.

The pay scale varies tremendously in this category. Promoters in large cities pay handsomely for many of these jobs—from $10 per hour to demonstrate a toy or a game to several hundred an hour to introduce a status item. If you become associated with a company that is doing continual promotions, you could become exclusively their employee and get their insurance, pension plan, etc.

SEVENTH AVENUE MODELING

Seventh Avenue in New York City is known for being the center of production of all the clothing made in America. It is not the only place where ready-to-wear clothing is manufactured in the United States, but it is the largest area of its kind. Everything from lingerie to fur coats is produced by these businesses, and Seventh Avenue models are required to wear the different garments when the buyers are in town.

A Seventh Avenue model must be a "model size," which varies according to who the designer is. Lingerie houses need fuller busts and longer legs, dress manufacturers want tall models (usually a size ten), and furriers look for slender models with broad shoulders so that the weighty furs hang well and look elegant.

This can be one of the tougher spots for a model to work. The people who run the huge garment houses are not known for their genteel manners, are extremely busy and often downright brusque. You must learn to take this in stride if you intend to start out in the garment district. The pressure is always at a maximum. Work is seasonal, and when you are hired by one of Seventh Avenue's showrooms, you really work for your pay.

There are differing opinions as to the value of showroom work as a jumping off point to a career in the modeling world, but working for a place that has fashion shows (or does them in conjunction with another showroom) can be beneficial. Fashion shows give you experience with runway work that you might not be able to get in New York without experience. Sometimes several houses combine for these shows, and you can make more suitable contacts for your climb up the modeling ladder.

Because the work is only seasonal, you don't have a long-term work commitment in an unexciting spot. Many clothes are designed on you, and that can be exciting—being part of the creative end. You may be offered some of the garments at almost cost to the manufacturer; it is a great way to have a unique wardrobe, as many of the samples are never mass-produced. Seventh Avenue modeling should not be viewed as a modeling career in itself. Few people can take the pressure continuously, and most want to try other fields of modeling as soon as possible.

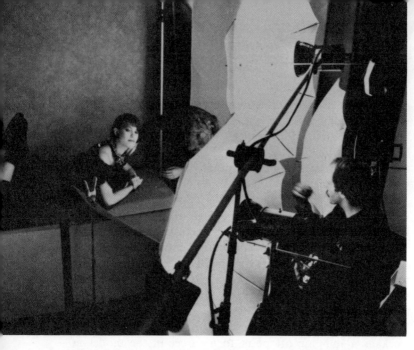

The photographer and assistant work together with the model to create a particular effect.

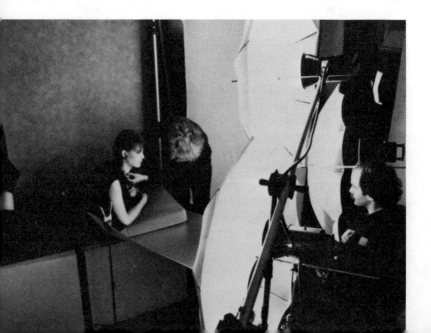

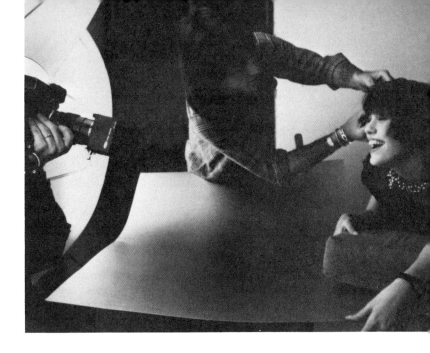

Photos: Renzo Renzi.

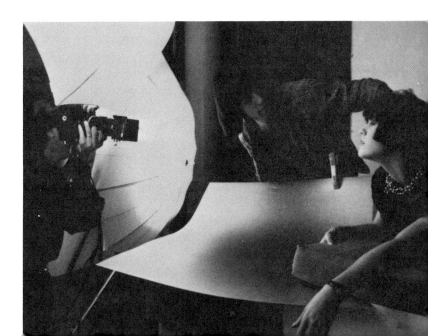

PHOTOGRAPHIC MODELING

Photographic modeling is perhaps the most well-known type of modeling. Men, women, and children comprise this group. The most famous is the high fashion model who appears in magazines, newspapers, promotional flyers, and on television and billboards. Men do not often do high fashion, so this is an area where ladies excel. Not only do women get most of the jobs, but they get the highest salaries as well.

At the bottom of the photographic scale, men and women have comparable incomes per job. As the woman ascends the fashion ladder, however, the demand is greater, the clothing more opulent, and the wage scale equable. After you have climbed slightly and your face becomes recognized by a few important clients, you (or your agency) will be able to command a higher hourly wage.

In high fashion, one of the most sought-after looks is one that portrays sultriness or classiness. Most models do not come from monied backgrounds, but every once in a while someone from royalty, or from a very wealthy family, tries her hand at high fashion work. This says something for the fun involved in women's fashion. Of course it is the rich and the royal who not only can afford high fashion, but also are the trendsetters in the fashion world. They are the audience at most of the shows, so fashion is a social event as well as big business. When the rich and famous do fashion work, it creates an aura of prestige over the industry.

A few years ago, the rich and famous all had every dress designed for them. Today, the richest of women buy their clothing ready-made, with only a few alterations as needed. By showing a finished costume with all its accessories, it is not unusual to sell an outfit in its entirety. Therefore the photographic model must appear to be comfortable as well as luxurious—not an easy task when you may actually be modeling this complete wool ensemble in steamy New York in the heat of August and you must look as though you are the lady of the manor greeting November!

Almost all photographic models are very tall. The male model in photographic work is often a sports celebrity, has far from perfect skin, and is not overly tall. It really is almost a one-on-one as to what is required for each shot. The general rule of thumb is that the person doing the modeling is in fairly good proportion and must be slender.

There is another whole area of photographic work wherein "real" people are employed. These are the models that you see having their cars repaired by other "mechanics" (models) in a little scenario played out in commercials. Though all models are known as "types," "real people" are a section unto themselves, and we will discuss that in a later chapter.

Photographic models are supposed to be the envy of every man and woman. The aura of this work is based on the premise that these are the chosen, the beautiful people. The psychology of modeling is sometimes a barrier difficult to surmount. Many people handle the job as just that; others are put off by its artificiality and as a result cannot "sell" themselves.

As in any other field, you must know yourself, what it is that will fulfill you and where you are headed. Thousands of people model to make money and then use the funds to accomplish other goals. Even a temporary career in modeling can make you a sizable nest egg, and even the best models do not last in the field much longer than five to seven years.

FASHION SHOW AND RUNWAY MODELING

High fashion work for a model could include several areas of the field. An extremely tall woman with a willowy body and very long legs is the epitome of the high fashion industry. Many years ago, the French were the whole center of this world. *Haute Couture* was all the rage. Names like Chanel, Saint Laurent, Dior, and Patou were on the lips of everyone who lived for fashion.

The fashion shows of Paris were (and a few still are) the more prestigious social events of the year. Collections were as guarded as the most expensive art treasures in the world. No one dared to leak a single clue to the press before the shows actually were staged and "stunned" the fashion world with the "new" look that would be expected to take the lead in what everyone would wear.

Runway models are usually quite stunning. Their main purpose is to look absolutely flawless to the naked eye. The model is selected to show off the garment to its best. She must make the beholder believe that the garment is elegant, feminine, chic, unique, alluring, a show-stopper, and expensive. Her presentation of the clothing is what modeling is all about. As an observer looks at the model, that potential customer's desire to be glamourous must be paramount. Very few women are nearly six feet tall and weigh less than 120 pounds. The trick here is to make the buyer think that she will look as great as the model does, and this does work!

Thousands of women buy fashions that a model has shown to rave reviews. So your job as the runway model is to endow the garment with such desirous qualities that its possession is critical to the audience. This is accomplished not only by the draping on a lanky frame, but by clever movements of the models that are choreographed to please the patrons. The current mode of motivation is a swagger. This motion can be observed on every video and movie of runway models at work. You will have to learn to move in all types of garments, and some of them are really designed to trip you up. One current trend is endless yards of fabric in one costume, and you have to learn to carry the bulk without making it look half as awkward as it really is. You will obviously look better in certain styles than others, but preference must never show: you're there to give your best to each garment.

It would be unusual to see a female model under six feet tall in a high fashion show, or one who weighed more than 120 pounds. Beauty is paramount for female models. Perfect features, small and straight, are required, and good hair is a must. Some exotic models are hired and regardless of their countries of origin do very well in all arenas of high fashion showing, the United States, France, Japan, and others.

You may not know if you could do this kind of work, but there are agency people who will be able to look you over and see your potential. It is often a woman who feels gangly, unattractive, and sometimes even the ugly duckling who blossoms into the incredible runway star. It is not easy to feel comfortable towering over your friends and family. When the skinny kid is polished into a fashion model, no one is more awestruck than the girl herself. So if you see a beanpole in your mirror, with tiny features and long, lanky legs, don't discount them as ugly. They may make you a very handsome income as a model.

Men in Fashion

There are some men in runway work now, as men's fashions have taken a swing into the luxury price brackets.

Designers use men to work their shows. Most of the men look like they are having a fairly good time. The fashions tend to be pretty casual compared to those worn by the women. Male models for these shows are supposed to exude a cross between understated sexy glances and suave appeal.

The high-priced clothing world for men has opened shows and the accompanying video work to men. These models are not exceptionally tall nor unlike each other; a standard size 40 suit would be a good measuring gauge.

TELEVISION MODELING

There are no set types for tv models. There are babies promoting diapers, ethnic groups pitching their favorite foods, celebrities pushing perfume, famous actors vouching for a variety of wines, high fashion models extolling the glories of department store furs, children eating tons of chocolates, and even the elderly demonstrating new sneakers or telephones! And everybody is dying to do television commercials simply because the pay is great and residuals are often greater than the pay for hourly modeling.

When you see famous sport stars and incredibly wealthy movie actors and actresses pushing products on tv, you know that they are really making good money for their time! The everyday person seen scrubbing a floor with a new soap product is not paid so handsomely, but the going rate of the tv commercial is still not paltry.

The qualifications are so widely varied that no one should be discouraged, but you should know that it is not just the "look" alone. Those who are seen, and those who are both seen and heard, comprise the two halves of tv modeling. There is one very good reason to be in the second category, as the pay scale doubles when the model speaks. But many people cannot do talking commercials. A baby may be too young or too independent to follow a script. Stage fright can simply make an otherwise stoic being crumble to bits. Many people simply have unpleasant voices.

Children who are selected to do tv work are picked because of their forwardness. An attack of shyness could blow a $10,000 commercial and more than a few clients.

There is always a need for specialty acts in tv commercials. Riding horses, jumping dirt bikes, sky diving, white water canoeing, or dancing exceptionally well could help you land that valuable job. There are hundreds of thousands of qualified people who could get the spot, but that little extra ability or unique talent may make the difference.

We have all sat through endless television ads of bodiless legs, hands, and teeth. These are owned by models who are unusually perfect in certain parts of their bodies. You could have a perfect profile and make an incredible income doing specialty work with that one feature. There are people with spectacular eyes who do commercials for everything from eye drops to the latest eye makeup. So if you feel that this area of tv might hold a place for you, investigate the modeling agencies who handle specialty models.

Don't negate a possibility! Prat falls and tossing pizzas could make you a nice little income in a tv commercial.

VIDEO MODELING

Video modeling is a fairly new area of the modeling field. A few years ago, movies were the only way of preserving the happenings at the prestigious high fashion shows in Paris. With the advent of video, many films are made and shown throughout the fashion world. These films include not only fashion openings, but the designer's full lines of clothing available to various shops and boutiques, closeup work of the high fashion makeup for these collections, and what the "look" is going to consist of for the season.

Video cameras can give wonderful coverage of all the major fashion shows throughout the world with a mere reloading of the equipment. Most department stores employ videos to advertise everything from electronic equipment to baked goods. The expansion of this type of communication has created thousands of jobs where there were only a handful before.

When you come across a real bottleneck in your favorite department store, you can be pretty sure that it is caused by fascinated video viewers craning to get a glimpse of the film. In New York City, there are literally hundreds of these machines throughout the stores, and they are always great eye-catchers. The advertiser knows just how to organize and package these films to entice the prospective customer to watch as though glued to the set. This fascination has been used to its fullest by advertisers. Models are paid thousands of dollars to move eternally on videotapes. The little machines keep rolling, and a show that in reality lasted approximately half an hour can now last forever. By paying the model to do a show that is videotaped, a designer's line can be shown to endless audiences, not limited to the physical capacity of the "houses" where the collection is originally presented.

The video camera, like the tv camera, is often cruelly unflattering to the model. Though a model may be absolutely breathtaking in person, the camera could distort her very badly. Since most high fashion show models are only seen by those of us not attending the original presentation, we must rely on the video's interpretation of what was seen. Therefore, though the runway model never used to have to be concerned with an ability to photograph well, that is seldom the case now.

Video modeling for commercials is very similar to modeling for television commercials in that the model is expected to talk, demonstrate, or visually endorse a variety of products. These videos could be strictly ads and can incorporate anyone who would or could be a television model from baby upward. Some tapes are used in an instruction capacity for the salesmen of a product to learn the pitch, as an eye-catching method to introduce a new product, or perhaps as a miniclip to be used educationally.

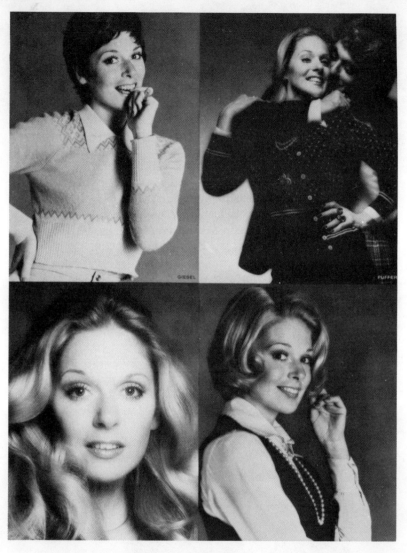

The composite should show off the versatility of the model, as in this page used by model Sandie Wolsfeld. Photo: Chic, Inc.; photographers Giesel and Puffer.

CHAPTER 2

QUALIFICATIONS NEEDED FOR THE VARIOUS MODELING JOBS

GENERAL ATTITUDE AND DRESS

The primary qualification needed for all types of modeling is the undying desire to be a model. Modeling is an extremely difficult field to break into. Few people are "discovered" and immediately enjoy the pleasures of the weekly pay check and real financial security. Most aspiring models have to "sell" themselves daily.

As a "new face," you are guaranteed bottom ranking in any modeling agency. You have to work every day by being available for endless "go-sees." No one is just going to hand you a job; you've got to be out there promoting yourself, and the more often your agency sends you the better your chances of establishing notoriety. You want to build up your name and visual profile as soon as possible, because agencies become quickly disenchanted with any model who is not putting forth lots of effort. If you are never available, frequently call in sick, or just have other things on your agenda, it won't be long before you find yourself without an agent.

Keep your eye on your goal. If you are rejected on a go-see, don't take it personally. If you never made the effort to get there, that's a different story. Your agency will keep trying for your probationary period just as long as you do. Even the most gorgeous person alive doesn't become a model instantly. Hard work derived from your innermost desire to be a model is the only way to make it.

A professional attitude toward yourself and your work is the next criterion. There are few other professions where you are so completely representing the marketable product (in this case *you*) *in total*. The client, your agency, the photographers, and even the stylists *will* be looking and remembering. You need to be remembered for that next job and future jobs. It is of paramount importance that you are remembered for being a pleasure to work with in every way. This means being physically appealing, neat, immaculately clean, and clean shaven (ladies and men), and having impeccable hair and nails. Many jobs are lost by models who are simply careless about personal care. When a model is not absolutely fastidious about cleanliness, it's one of those situations where an employer or client will not call the person for a job ever again.

Clean and neat clothing from undergarments outward are a real boon. One male model states that (early in his career) he was made very aware that agents as well as clients were scrutinizing his garments as part of his total appearance. The call-backs that he has received have proven him to be right. Even if you don't have an extensive wardrobe, be certain that you appear in fresh looking garments, of as good quality as you can possibly afford.

With all the current advertising emphasis on designers' names, you will want to own clothing that is recognizable as chic to those whom you are trying to impress. It's not a must that you have any identifying labels. You must demonstrate your fashion awareness by a generally "in" look or costume. Observe other models' get-ups as they dress for go-sees. There is such a wide variance in self-sell modes that once you are a little more sure of your placement in the modeling agency, you are a bit freer to set differing looks for different jobs. Models (known and not so well established) can be seen on their way to jobs in New York in everything from really ratty jeans to exquisite suits with a full complement of accessories. Both ends of the fashion spectrum are worn by models. The correct timing is the all-important key to when it's right to wear what.

What is really unique to New York is the personal mix of what amounts to fashion. Mink and blue jeans, evening gowns and vintage wraps, casual and formal wear in one costume are all part of the current fashion scene, so you are pretty much able to "do it yourself," as long as the final creation is within a certain arena. That arena changes rapidly and the really avant garde always have the most fun with clothing. In fashion, you can't be a follower, and if you get too far ahead of the pack, you're just that. Keep a keen eye on the current fashion trends, and *try* to dress as you will be expected to as a representative of the fashion world.

PHYSICAL QUALIFICATIONS
FOR HIGH FASHION

First on the list is *youth*! Many high fashion models as young as thirteen years of age are involved in career modeling. Their annual incomes rank among the highest salaries paid to any workers, including corporate executives, doctors, and attorneys. These very young ladies are the beauties whose figures and faces are seen daily in publications and on television. All of them are between the ages of perhaps even 11 to 23. The really great high fashion model can stretch her career into her middle to late twenties if she is very lucky. That is truly an unusual phenomenon though, so the earlier you start, the better your chances at making a career in this field.

The second qualification is that your height must be somewhere between five feet, eight inches and six feet tall. A really stunning beauty at five feet, seven and a half inches could get by. The idea here is proportionate height with very slender limbs. So, if you are extremely fine boned though shorter, you might still have a chance at high fashion work.

Weight is critical. You cannot weigh more than 125 pounds, and that would be on the tallest frame. Most of the models weigh around 115 to 120. Your weight has to stay consistent. This is accomplished by sticking to a highly restricted diet and exercise.

The weight must be distributed proportionately over your frame. You must not have any bulges or even any visible bumps. Long and slender is the guide. Arms, legs, torso, and neck should be as lean as the proverbial race horse. The bust is usually not larger than a B cup, but you could look into lingerie work if you are larger. Long, lanky, and nicely-shaped legs are critical. Much of fashion depends on the height of the model and how the garment looks on the over-tall frame. The desired spot to carry the extra height is in the leg, not the torso or neck.

Another important characteristic is that you must have a very photogenic face. This usually means straight features that are rather small. If you want to do runway work exclusively, you need not worry about being photogenic, but most models in the high fashion category combine all the areas possible to round out their careers, as well as their incomes. If you have some snapshots that look pretty bad, don't assume that you do not photograph well. It may be that all you need is a good professional photographer who will take the time to work with you. Few models photograph the way they really look. The camera can lie, and it's not a sure bet in which way! Sometimes an incredible beauty looks almost ugly and vice versa.

Your face can make a tremendous difference not only in your potential income but in your total life as a model. The right combination of attractive eyes, alignment of nose and alluring mouth could be the difference between an average model and a million dollar one.

Look in the mirror and honestly assess what you see. Make-up does help tremendously, but the bottom line basics are the aforementioned, plus no visible marks. If you have any scars, beauty marks, heavy freckles, or real variance in structure, they could be against you. Some freckles are considered to be very much in vogue, particularly in cases where the model is endowed with gorgeous red hair and golden or blue to green eyes.

Trying to change your physical attributes through plastic surgery is possible but advisable only if you are genuinely unhappy with your face—perhaps a small scar or mark. Modeling can be extremely fickle. What is "in" today could be as unpopular next month as the flu. Many times a model has been advised to have rhinoplasty only to have a worse nose afterward or to discover that the original is now what is in style. Noses with bumps in the bridge, bushy eyebrows, slightly crooked smiles, irregular jaw lines, and ill-matched eyes are just a few of the trendy flaws that come and go in fashion work. Don't outguess the agents; what you consider an imperfection they may be able to turn into a desirable characteristic.

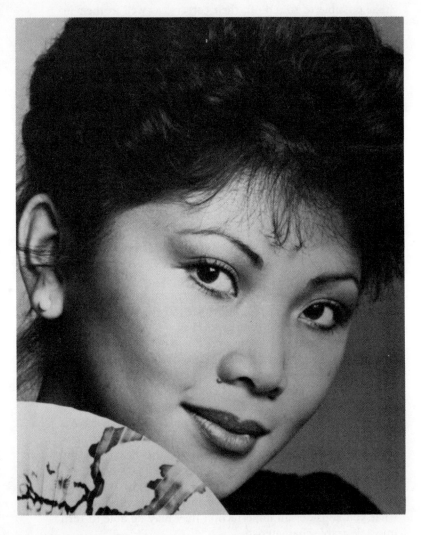

Model Ermenilda uses this shot to emphasize eyes and other features. Photo: Chic, Inc.

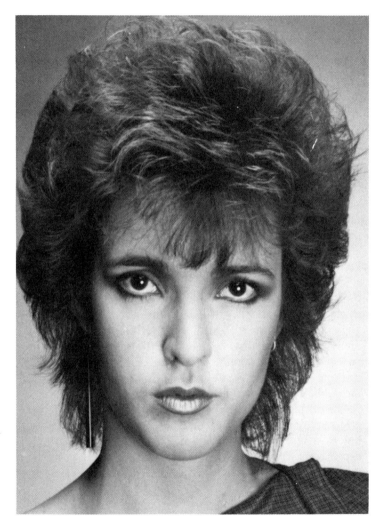

Head-on shot emphasizes symmetry, line, and balance of features. Photo: Pivot Point.

Hair, teeth, and skin must be healthy, attractive, and vibrant. An all-round complement of appealing good looks is critical.

Some high fashion designers seek out a certain "look" for their collections, a look that is instantly recognizable for their particular lines or collections. If you look at the fashion spreads, you will be able to see at a glance what style is developed by each designer. Some are enchanted with the classic beauty, with fair hair and skin, light eyes, small tipped-up nose, and a generally English countryside appearance. Other designers prefer sultry brunettes to carry off the look of their collections. It is the complete impression of the coloring and facial expression of the high fashion model that is sought after for much live and photographic work.

Different modeling agencies actually "specialize" in these various looks, and the largest agencies are able to supply everything from cute to sultry-looking models, depending on the client's needs. Some newer models try to develop a single "look" that they will be known for. Others are as wide-ranging in their "look" as a chameleon; you would really not believe that it could be the same person from page to page in a layout. Clever makeup, hair styles, and clothing can and do create totally different presentations to the public's eye.

The different looks that you will be required to create are affected by not only the costume, makeup, and scenery, but by a mood you communicate through facial and body expressions. The most clever models are good at mime; they can represent an action, character, mood, or feeling by imitation. Some articles of clothing lend themselves to a certain feeling on the part of the model. Imagination is critical, as there are often situations where you are handed an item and expected to wing it.

Movement is an asset for the would-be model, as there isn't an easy way to learn the actions needed by the fashion world without a little innate grace and skillful emulation. Opinions differ as to the easiest way to acquire the necessary agility. Rhythm does not come easily to everyone, so the earlier that you become engaged in some kind of dance, sports, or music, the easier the art of moving well and with confidence will develop. If you have poise and self-assurance, moving like a high fashion model will be simple enough to learn. But if you have to start from the very beginning even to have ease of movement, you could be in trouble. Even as a young adult, poor carriage and stilted motions are a giveaway that you are really ill at ease, and this is a profession where your basic job is to convey absolute self-confidence.

To have the winning combination of desire, great looks, height, slenderness, poise, beauty of face and proportionate figure, and youth is to be in possession of the right physical characteristics for a high fashion model. There are, of course, emotional and professional characteristics required as well. These are discussed elsewhere in this book.

SPECIFIC QUALIFICATIONS FOR ALL MODELS

Physical good health is paramount for modeling. The stress can be intense, the hours brutal, the positions difficult, the travel wearing, and the weather trying for outdoor work. If you don't feel in top-notch shape, you're simply not going to last as long as you're required to, and exhaustion will cost everyone from your agency to the client.

Discipline is rigid for every model, children included. You must keep a consistent weight, build, and all around

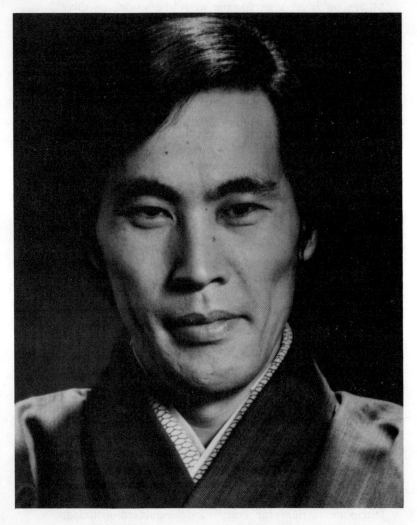

Actor and model Kensuke Haga in traditional Japanese dress. Photo: SWG.

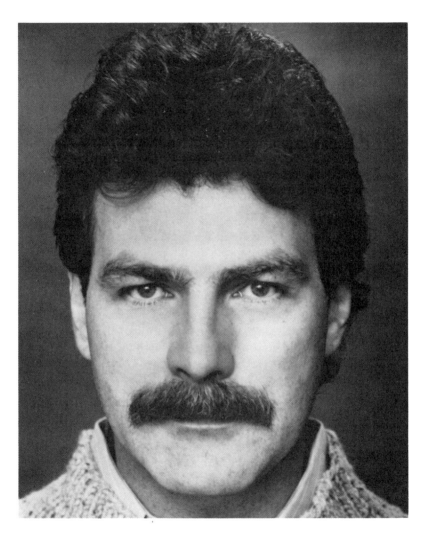

Model Richard Feenstra in sportswear. Photo: SWG.

"look." Your diet and exercise regimen must be strictly followed and eight hours of sleep is critical for you to look and perform well.

Patience is a virtue you will need every time you have an interview, a go-see, or a session. Sometimes there are delays and hitches that make you want to scream. Keep calm. Hysterics will make you an instantly unpopular model, and the others who can hold up under pressure will be the ones asked for return engagements. There is nothing worse than helping to make a bad situation a disaster, so try to remain cool while others lose their tempers. You'll be remembered and rewarded.

Enthusiasm makes the really great models. Sprightly young models are the mainstay of the business and promote everything from foods to bobby pins, with an effervescent quality that often appears to be genuine. It has been said by agents that the person with the greatest charm, sparkle, and passion can compete successfully with the greater natural beauty who lacks fire.

You must be able to take rejection as a daily diet without getting depressed. Every time you are sent on a go-see, the chances are that you only "may" get that job. Many people compete for each one. You must keep a permanently optimistic view toward your career and yourself. This is the hardest part for many models, because rejection just does make you feel discouraged. You have to keep trying and trying and trying. That seventh or eighth go-see just may be the plum that you've prayed for.

You need an endless ability to take criticism and work with it. You may be asked or even rudely told to do something like hold a very difficult pose. For all of your serious endeavors, it may not work. After agonizing for some time, the tempers begin to flare. You, as the model, are the target, and you simply have to keep trying to get it right. Criticism is the only way the photographer is able to elicit the best shots, and if you're not an instantaneous "natural" (and about one in a million is "at home" in front of camera, photographer, and stylists all demanding at once), then you have to give a thousand per cent every time you are asked to do a job. The cooperation of everyone is really visible in the final product.

You will be well-advised to have a sense of humor. Things can and do go wrong. A sense of humor can relieve the tension so that progress can be resumed.

You must keep yourself organized. This means being fully prepared for every job promptly, enthusiastically, and professionally. You can *never* be late to a go-see or an actual job! That is an unforgivable transgression. It keeps an entire group of people (who are getting paid) waiting, and you may never see another job through your agency again. Everyone has a schedule to meet, and your major responsibility is to get there on time! Excuses are unacceptable in this trade. If you are genuinely ill or there is a real crisis, you are expected to call your agency at the earliest moment so that the fewest people will be inconvenienced by the change in schedule.

You will be expected to be congenial and yet not socialize. Everyone there is ready to work, and it is very difficult for some to realize that this is an atmosphere of serious and hard endeavor. You must not get carried away with the idea of being a star, but realize that this is primarily work and that if you let yourself slip into an unhealthy frame of mind, it could have some serious repercussions. One very successful, internationally known model says that it is quite common for new men and women to blow their whole potential career with their attitudes of superiority and subsequent lack of professionalism. They get caught up in the myth that models are glamourous and terrific, and they forget how replaceable they are. Many other models are waiting in the wings.

You must realize at this juncture that you will not be able to have a full social life. When all of your friends are ready to start the night's activities, you will be bowing out for an early night's sleep. When you are expected to look sensational at six in the morning, that means showing up looking rested and fresh, not haggard and with bags under your eyes. The only models who can get by with a normal social calendar are the television subjects for cold remedy and sleeping tablet commercials. Modeling is a difficult and highly disciplined way of life. Before choosing it, you should weigh the sacrifices against the rewards.

SPECIFIC QUALIFICATIONS
FOR THE MALE MODEL

Male modeling is coming into its own and can now be considered a true career area for men. A few years ago, the major work for the male model was work as a backup to the high fashion model, or catalog work. The field has expanded so much that most modeling agencies have opened sections for the men only. The criterion used to be the 40 regular suit. Now there is a little variation, though not too much in either direction. The main thing that the agencies are looking for in the male model is a really appealing face and slender body. The current look is very clean-cut collegiate, in variations of blond and brown hair.

Critical here is the photogenic requirement, as that is the basic bread-and-butter area for men. Runway modeling is a new field for men and though you might not need to be photogenic for that specific job, most runway work using male models is being videotaped. There is so little work for the male model that does not involve photography that he should not seriously consider a career in the field unless the camera is kind to him.

Agencies are looking for men between six feet and six feet, two inches tall who lend themselves to the "look" that the agencies represent. A fashion look is currently in vogue.

If you have the basic criteria, send a few snapshots to a local or even the largest agencies. If they think you have the potential, they'll advise you. Then if you are in the area, you'll want to set up an interview to confirm that what the agent needs, you have. The agency will then set about helping you to acquire really good photographs (testing) so that your pictures will fit the requirements. They will guide you and turn you into a polished model with the look that will be beneficial to both them and you.

The more unique facial features are most in demand. Look through men's fashion magazines and keep an eye on newspaper photographs of the current popular male models to give you an idea of the needed features, haircuts, bone structures, and coloring.

Pretty teeth, sparkling or sensual eyes, and a fairly straight nose are required. Smaller features are the most fashionable-looking. That lovely combination of perfect proportion in facial features and slender, tall body are the winning criteria for the male model.

Black and exotic male models are needed in all of the various areas of modeling. The ages of male models are more widespread than of the females. A man in the field could last from his teens through his forties as long as he maintained his good looks and his slender frame.

Catalogs have been known to show male models over a span of twenty years! One male model who is still working and is in his fifties looks as if he is in his mid-thirties. His self-discipline has been extraordinarily consistent, and it has paid off. He has been a professional male model for over thirty years and has made a very nice living with his chosen career.

SPECIFIC QUALIFICATIONS FOR CHILD MODELS

Children are used in modeling for catalogs, television, and print ads. Child models are required to be very well behaved and cooperative. As they are working and are being paid for such, though you cannot expect adult behavior, absolute complaisance is critical. Child models must be unique, charming, appealing, cute, or pretty. They must be a perfect size. They must be photogenic, and they must want to work. It's not enough that they have all of the potential, unless they themselves want to model.

The pay scale is enough to make any parent consider the prospects, but the child's the one who will be doing the sitting, so make sure that he or she really wants to work. If you have a child that you think might make a good model, send snapshots to an agency in your area, and they will get back to you if they are interested. Be sure to include a letter telling the child's statistics: clothing and shoe sizes, age, hair and eye coloring (if shots are black-and-white), height, and weight.

A Word of Caution to Parents

If you are considering a modeling career for your child, be sure to write to your local labor department for any work permits required by your particular state. There are several other permits required by various groups to protect the child, and your agency will advise you of these.

If you or your child are considering a television commercial as a source of income, check with the various unions such as SAG (Screen Actors' Guild) and AFTRA (American Federation of Television and Radio Artists). You are only permitted to do your first commercial without membership in these unions.

SPECIFIC QUALIFICATIONS
FOR THE TELEVISION MODEL

Anyone *could* be a television model. That covers the entire gamut of physical characteristics from babies to grandmothers. The most often used models are young, pretty women who promote products. Aside from the high fashion model, whose criteria we discussed earlier, these women could be anywhere from petite to amazon in structure, and the men could be any look from the innocent little boy to the grumpy insomniac. The variations are endless!

There are two distinct parts of television modeling. You must be extroverted, determined, and self-assured to do the modeling, but you must also be capable of speaking for the media if you're going to be doing the talking as well. You'll want to take lessons if you can't make the second half of the criteria, as they're the ones who get paid doubly. There is no such thing as being a wrong type for tv work, it's merely a matter of waiting until the demand for your "look" comes along. There are people who are very talented and appear time and again in commercials. They develop different characters for every ad. These models are often professional actors who have the advantage of not only having a "look" but also a particular chameleon ability. If you are seriously considering tv work, try to do a little acting and then contact a local agency to see what kind of head shot they require and accompany it with your resumé at your interview.

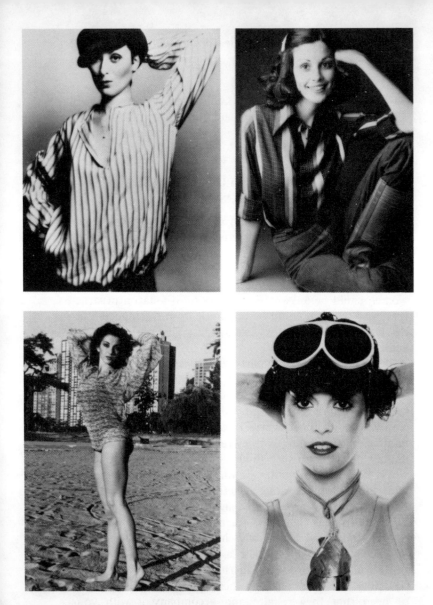

The composite should include a variety of poses, moods, and styles as in this one, above. Photo: Chic, Inc.

CHAPTER 3

HOW TO BREAK INTO MODELING

Ways to get started in the modeling world are as diversified as the number of jobs available. If you are certain of your potential qualifications at this point, then it will be a bit easier to determine your starting area. If you are very young, you will need all the encouragement and guidance that you can get.

HOW DO YOU KNOW IF
YOU HAVE WHAT IT TAKES?

If you live in an area away from major cities, you will have to rely on your own hunches and trying to establish yourself as being attractive in the local public eye. It is difficult without having the advantage of the professional's experience to judge, but you generally know if you feel that you might have the potential. That is the starting point.

If you've already been noticed by local photographers or been considered good-looking by others all your life, you are probably at least attractive. The only way to know what that might mean for you as a model is to proceed in the general direction of public affirmation of your physical attributes. Popularity must not be confused with possible modeling qualifications.

After you have read chapter one of this book, you should have a better idea where you fit in. The dictates are pretty clear-cut, so don't expect an agency to make exceptions. If your reflection shows you a short, rounded figure with hips and sloping shoulders, don't torture yourself by trying to be what you're not. There are millions of job opportunities in the world. If your heart's desire is to be in the modeling world, maybe you could be happy in a model-associated field. Or maybe you would be satisfied as a specialty model who has some perfect parts like hands, face, or smile. It is obviously more difficult to test the waters for your potential ability in rural areas. Your best bet might be to have some good photographs made of your hands or some good head shots and send them with a covering letter and a resume to an agency. If they are interested, they will make an appointment with you. Many modeling schools in smaller city areas are a good source of contact. When you take classes with them, it often entitles you to do regional modeling work.

You need lots of exposure to get a good handle on public response to your ability to model. The tinier the geographical area, the harder it will be to gain this kind of exposure, but there are endless ways to expand this limitation. After you have contacted the modeling schools, make an effort to write or talk to all the nearby cities with agencies. From there, you may want to enter all the local beauty contests and visit all the department stores and malls, leaving your name and photo (with your statistics and phone number). You may be surprised at the amount of work that can come your way in this manner. If a model is needed for a promotion, and you were clever enough to have left all the needed information, you will probably be the first chosen. It's happened more often than one would suppose that a "break" was prepared ahead of time by an aspirant and luck did the rest. There is just too much competition for these jobs for you to be able to sit back and wait for them to come to you.

Suppose you are doing all right in a medium-sized city as a model. You may be perfectly happy there and though the money is not earthshaking, you could make a decent living ($7,000 to $15,000, keeping quite busy with runway work, promotional work, photographic work, and whatever local television work that you could pick up). You are to be in demand and available full-time. If you are totally dependent upon your modeling wages, you could be left nearly penniless, so either make certain to have a nest egg to tide you over, or do modeling as a secondary job.

As a high fashion model hopeful, you will have to make your way to either New York City, Los Angeles, or Chicago. Two smaller cities with moderate amounts of work to offer would be Atlanta and Cleveland in the East, and San Francisco and Dallas in the West. You may want to give these cities a try before you feel confident enough to approach the capitals of modeling.

Any positive experience under your belt will be an added plus in your climb up the ladder in a modeling career.

THE BEAUTY CONTEST

Thousands of aspiring young women have entered local beauty pageants in the hope of being discovered as models, starlettes, and eventual celebrities. These contests are always open to pretty or talented girls. Some even include women who have grown children! There is so much chance for media coverage in these contests that even if you are not any more than a local winner, you could get quite a bit of mileage out of the publicity. There are also the added incentives of prizes and possible scholarships and contracts. It can be a surprisingly good stepping-stone.

Agents and their assistants have a keen eye focused on the many contests that occur annually. Many an ignored contestant has become a top model, partly because beauty pageants are geared toward a much meatier body than fashion modeling and partly because many beauty contestants photograph well but do not come across well in personal appearances (critical to the mass promotions on such contests). There is no longer a stigma on entering to win, and it is not unusual to see last year's Miss State XYZ be this year's representative of State ZYX, having established residency in the six months required to qualify. And amazingly, these women time and again walk off with the prizes the second, third, or even fourth time around. There is obviously something to be said for their methodical approaches.

Very few people would want to make a career of vying annually for places in beauty pageants, but as far as a lesson in persistence goes, it's somewhat the same attitude that you'll have to have with modeling. If you are convinced that you really want to get into modeling, there are hundreds of beauty contests available to you. Start by reading the magazines geared to the teenage market, and carefully select those contests that offer modeling jobs as prizes. There are many such contests, but the entry fees may be costly and the wardrobe another out-of-pocket expense. Some contests are so costly that sponsors are available, and you will have to investigate which ones will promote you the best toward your modeling goal.

A local pageant may give you the experience that will help you get to the top in a bigger one, or you may want to try for the nationals right away.

One major drawback in the two largest contests (Miss

America and Miss Universe) is the age to enter. If you are young and heart-set on a high fashion career, you may do better to give the smaller contests your attention, as they are geared to the teenagers exclusively. Youth being the marketable item that it is, you may be wasting precious time by holding out for bigger stakes.

The most well-known beauty contests for teenagers are given in the following list. It is best for you to write directly to each for information regarding the time, place, entry fees, and rules. So study the regulations and be aware of what they can do to help your career get started.

MISS TEENAGE AMERICA
'Teen Magazine
8490 Sunset Blvd.
Los Angeles, CA 90069

MISS AMERICAN TEENAGER, INC.
P.O. Box 221
New Milford, NJ 07646

NATIONAL TEENAGER
215 Piedmont Ave. N.E.
Atlanta, GA 30312

MISS TEEN U.S.A.
2250 North Druid Hills Rd. N.E.
Atlanta, GA 30329

MISS TEEN WORLD
1491 Hidden Hills Pkwy.
Stone Mountain, GA 30088

MISS TEEN ALL-AMERICA
Att: Syd Sussman
1220 East West Highway, Suite 101
Silver Springs, MD 20910

AMERICA'S JUNIOR MISS PAGEANT
P.O. Box 2786
Mobile, AL 36601

MISS BLACK AMERICA PAGEANT
24 W. Chelton Ave., Suite 202
Philadelphia, PA 19144

MISS WORLD-AMERICA PAGEANT
Griff O'Neil
500 E. 77th St., Suite 328
New York, NY 10021

MISS AMERICA PAGEANT
Boardwalk Arcade Building
Boardwalk and Tennessee Ave.
Atlantic City, NJ 08401

MISS U.S.A. PAGEANT and
MISS UNIVERSE PAGEANT
International Headquarters
Miss Universe, Inc.
640 Fifth Ave.
New York, NY 10019

The aforementioned contests can give you great exposure and lots of press coverage. With all the photography and television, you will be able to get an idea of how you look on film. There are many local contests that lead up to the bigger ones, and every inch of the way could help your modeling career along. As long as you hold even the most insignificant title, people are curious to see what and who you are, so don't hesitate to push yourself forward for even the smallest contests. Modeling is nothing but competition at the bottom line, and every chance to compete should be welcomed.

The more experience the better. The competition must be overcome in such a way that you come out on top looking like you were just the best choice, not clawing tooth and nail to push yourself to the forefront. Everything has been tried, from researching the judges' backgrounds (to better prepare answers that would please their interests), to extensive plastic surgery (in the hope of being just what the judges are looking for). You'll do best by sticking with what you already have. Beauty contests are judged by human beings whose ideas of beauty are often pretty wide-ranged. You could spend your entire life arranging yourself to suit someone else's likes or expectations.

Two other competitions in particular are conducted with a modeling contract offered as a prize. The most famous is "Face Of The 80's" (in association with Ford Models, Inc.), and the other is *'Teen's* Great Model Search.

"Face Of The 80's"

You can enter "Face Of The 80's" by filling out an application run in your local newspapers. The entry form must be accompanied by two snapshots of yourself (a head shot and a full length). Women between the ages of sixteen and twenty may enter, but you cannot have more than two years of modeling experience. You must be between five feet, eight inches and five feet, ten inches tall.

This contest has tremendous prestige in the modeling world. The prize is a modeling contract that puts you in line for all kinds of media exposure. The woman who wins "Face Of The 80's" is shot into the national spotlight immediately.

'*Teen's* Great Model Search

'*Teen's* Great Model Search also has a modeling contract prize. This competition is sponsored by the Gillette Company and offers a one-year modeling contract to the winner. To enter, you must be between the ages of twelve and eighteen, and desire to become a model. For more information write to Great Model Search, 'Teen Magazine, P.O. Box 69940, Los Angeles, CA 90069.

HEADING STRAIGHT FOR THE BIG AGENCIES

If you already live in or near New York, Chicago, or Los Angeles, you may want to approach the top people in the field. The big agencies are naturally where the largest amounts of money are to be made, and if you are truly qualified, why shouldn't you start at the highest salary that you can command?

Call and make an appointment with an interviewer. Some agencies prefer that you bring photographs so that the interviewer can see how photogenic you are. If you only have bad shots of yourself and you realize that they are awful, *don't take them* to an agent. The scrutinizing eye of the agent will be able to tell whether you should invest in *any* shots. They might not be interested at all, and then you would be wasting your money and time. On the other hand, if you have good photographs of your face and full body, you will certainly want to show them to the agent. The agent will be looking at how well your bone structure comes across on a photograph.

The interviewers' keen eye is really critical in delineation of potential models. Their experience in what to look for can save you many hours of indecision. If you are just what that particular agency needs, you may happily end your search. If not, you must make another and another appointment until you have exhausted all of the agencies, large and small, that you would consider working for.

Give yourself a fair chance to get into an agency. After several months and some polishing of your whole look, however, if you are still pounding the sidewalks, start to think of another profession. The experts really do know and there's very little that can be done to change the current selling look.

BREAKING INTO TELEVISION MODELING

Many models are already working as photographic models when they make the first step into the television commercial. Such people are guided by their agents and are prepared for the audition so that they know what to expect. An audition of any kind can be a pretty awful experience, and it is particularly noted for its ego-destruction. Of course if you *do* land the part, you can feel really elated. Your agent will guide you as to what looks best on film vis-a-vis your mode of dress, the actual pattern of your clothing, your color scheme, and the kind of clothes that your portrayed character is supposed to be wearing. Your makeup and hair will also have to be suited to the character role. Try to feel comfortable with your costume, so that you can concentrate on the critical part of the audition.

You will arrive at the audition site at the scheduled time, tell the receptionist that you are there, and then wait, nervously sizing up the competition. You will have brought your resume and your head shot, which you will leave for the casting director to review or merely to remind him who (of the thousands) you were.

(of the thousands) you were.

After a while, you will be introduced to other models who may be sharing this commercial with you. You will also be given your script and told the general story line of what will be acted in your little scenario. You may or may not have a speaking part. If you do speak, you will have to memorize your lines, and then the cues and directions.

Suppose you are trying for a hair product commercial. Directors usually look for blondes, because highlights are more easily picked up when the hair is light, and because the United States is a blonde-oriented society. Semi-long hair has more movement to it and is considered to be more sensual. If you have both the right color and length, your chances are greatly improved. Your next problem is to move with ease and be completely relaxed with a television camera, crew, a whole room full of strangers, and your mini-skit jiggling around in your head.

Having gotten this far, you are ready to go in front of the cameras. Things seldom go as planned. You may find yourself doing not one but as many as a dozen or more takes. If there are more people involved in the commercial, it could take quite a while just to coordinate everyone. Trying to make each take seem fresh and natural is easier said than done. Take number one may be stiff, but by the time you get to take number fifteen, exhaustion will have overcome stiffness.

If you can develop the knack of doing television commercials, the thousands of dollars plus residuals paid for each one more than compensate for the boredom, anxiety, cattle-call degradation, and myriad takes.

After successfully getting through one of these little commercial vignettes, you may consider doing another one. Viewers automatically assume that if a person endorses a product (models with it or promotes it verbally), that person surely *uses* it as well. This is often just not the case, but the manufacturer of the product that you have promoted does have the right to prevent you from modeling for that company's direct competitors for a period of time (depending on the contract you signed). If you modeled for a certain company's new color-rinse shampoo and then were offered a commercial by another hair product company to model their anti-dandruff shampoo, the advertisers would see that as a definite conflict of interest. You would have to turn down the second company's offer. You could, however, do any unrelated area of products from any non-shampoo-making company.

If you don't land that first commercial, try again. If you feel that your hair is your best asset, try for all the endless hair accessories, hair dryers, shampoos, rinses, dyes, clippers, pins, gels, curling irons, hair pieces, treatments, medications, highlighters, curlers, home permanents, and even stylists' commercials. Competition is fierce, but perseverence can pay off. Many models have started their careers with a hair commercial and then been noticed for the whole person from that angle.

Unions

Unions strictly protect people who perform the commercials, according to pay scale, time allowed to work, and where and when work can be done. When you try for your first commercial you will not need to worry about this stipulation; you are permitted one "free" commercial before you are forced to join a union (or unions). The union sets a uniform pay scale that must be strictly adhered to regardless of the person's status as model, actor, or even person- off-the-street. All ages of people are included in these codes. Your agent can advise you as to which unions to join, and where and how to pay your annual dues.

There are two unions that you may need to join if you intend to do extensive work in television commercials. One covers live commercials, and the other covers videotaped commercials:

AFTRA
(American Federation of Television and Radio Artists)
1350 Avenue of the Americas
New York, NY 10019

SAG (Screen Actors Guild)
1700 Broadway
New York, NY 10001

There are rules as to which union coverage you will have to have. Lacking an agent, you must be responsible for your own protection. That means inquiring and applying for these union memberships as needed.

Membership in the American Federation of Television and Radio Artists (AFTRA) is currently $600 and annual dues are $28.75 semiannually. AFTRA is an open union.

Membership in the Screen Actors Guild (SAG) is currently $637.50 and annual dues are $75.

To apply for membership to the Guild, you must have done anything under SAG's jurisdiction (such as a screen feature film or commercial), or have been a member of one of the following for at least a year:

AEA (Actors' Equity Association)
AFTRA (American Federation of Television and Radio Artists)
AGMA (American Guild of Musical Artists)
AGVA (American Guild of Variety Artists)
Hebrew Actors' Union
Italian Actors' Union

Resume

A resume is very important if you are planning to audition for television commercials. The resume should give all the critical statistics. A particular style or layout, clever arrangement of the critical information, or artistic touches may help you catch the employer's eye. The most important thing is to remember that your resume's function is to include all of the pertinent data and make a neat impression. Therefore, the first section must include your name, address, and phone number (or your answering service, manager, or agent).

The next section should include your social security number and your union associations and membership numbers.

The following division should include your physical data: height, weight, hair color, eye color, and your general look or type. Include the age range that you *could* honestly portray. Your clothing sizes should be listed—for a suit, shirt, shoe, hat, and gloves if you are a man; and for a hat, dress, shoe, glove, and undergarments and swimwear if you are a woman. Most women are more detailed in the department of measurements. You may want to be explicit as to bust, waist, and hip measurements.

As you will be promoting your vocal abilities if you intend to talk (and talking in any commercial doubles your pay scale) in your audition and subsequently in commercials, you will want to mention the level of your voice (tenor, for example) and the list of any movies or commercials you've done. Mention any live theater productions and the parts you acted. Give all the correct information about each theatrical production and where and when it was performed.

If you were coached by someone of renown, list it clearly

under *Professional or Special Training.* Also indicate any dance training, fencing, competitive sports, or any other type of movement instruction that could indicate agility or skilled grace. Mention any kind of unusual talent—like sky diving, scuba diving, windsurfing, sailing, skiing, diving, ice skating, horseback riding, pizza tossing, whistling.

The ability to speak any foreign languages should be noted, and your own nationality and native tongue if it is not simply North American. Even variations in United States accents can make or break your chances at the job.

One last thing to include in your resume is the name of a reference or two if you are not being represented by an agent upon introduction.

Your resume is most often typed on a sheet of paper that fits against and is firmly attached to your glossy eight-by-ten photograph, back to back. Nothing says that you have to fill up your eight-by-ten resume, but do center the information. Neatness and professionalism count a great deal. If you value your crack at the commercial, make your photograph and your resume attractively displayed and appealing.

The photograph that is so important is supposed to be a lively image with projection. The old high school graduate shot is considered to be too stiff and certainly won't get you past the casting agent. There is such a prescribed definitive look that you have to spend a good bit of time on this project. More often than not, your idea of how you look best is *not* their idea of your best shot! They want to see how you will come across as a warm, believable, likable person. This is not an easy request of one sample photograph.

After much stewing and brewing in front of a photographer who specializes in head shots for television commercial hopefuls, you may come up with one or even two passable shots. Try to get another professional opinion about which shots are best for you. The expense of these head shots will be $500 to $1000, depending on your choice of photographer and how many prints you decide to have made. This can be a rather large investment if you are doing many auditions and you leave the photograph with attached resume with the casting directors of each. But this photograph can be the reminder that could and often has secured a future or even a different job than the one you tried for.

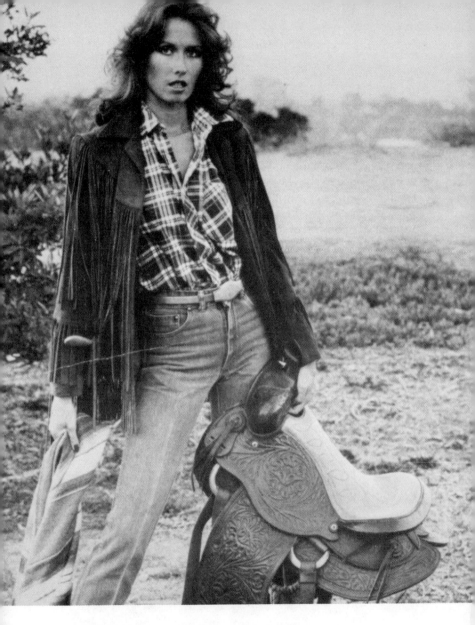

Model Joan E. Harris in Western dress, Photo: Chic, Inc.

CHAPTER 4

PREPARATION FOR BECOMING A MODEL

IS MODELING SCHOOL NEEDED?

Modeling schools are actually establishments that give courses in a wide variety of subjects, from poise and makeup to vocal lessons and how to "sell" yourself. The many different types of modeling opportunities available have caused the charm school market to expand greatly.

Some of the know-how transmitted includes how to work in front of cameras, how to work with photographers, how to move on runways for fashion work, how to do your own makeup for modeling jobs, and how to present yourself.

A modeling or charm school prepares you to handle situations that may arise in any modeling assignment. You do actual makeup, hairstyles, and even wardrobe articles on yourself to learn the tricks of the trade. You learn how to diet, exercise, and keep an eye on your figure. Instruction is given in how to carry yourself and move with a sense of style. Various types of modeling require certain turns, walks, and posturing. A school has all of the physical setups that emulate the real thing to give you experience with those situations and circumstances.

Familiarity with how you appear on film and video can give you insight into your potential future in the varied areas of modeling. Mock-ups of actual "shows" will prepare you for work with commentators as timing is an essential in this work. Every modeling situation will be different, but the more aware you are of what may occur, the more confident you may feel.

There are modeling schools in every major city where you could inquire as to the courses given, the time allotted, and the cost. Some of the schools are strictly charm instruction and will simply give the student a little polish. In really rural areas, exposure to the self-improvement courses is valuable simply as an introduction to basic fashion.

In very small towns, modeling work is generally limited to department store shows and social events where models might be the entertainment for a ladies group. The school may work as a small agency and may or may not collect a fee to arrange these modeling shows. But the model is usually compensated in some way and at the very least is gaining experience and exposure to the public.

The reason for attending any school is to learn to do something that you did not know how to do beforehand. There are many hundreds of people who have all the raw qualities mentioned in Chapter 2. For people who already have great self-assurance and all the needed physical attributes, attending modeling school would be superfluous.

A modeling agency that wants to put you under contract though you are completely inexperienced will undertake your training or see to any needed instruction. Many agencies see to your development in a European arena because the photographers are better known for taking the time to work with a very young and inexperienced model.

With European training, it is easier to land the higher paying jobs in the United States. Some models become enamored with not only the modeling work in Europe, but with the lifestyle there. For many, what started as an education in a new field turned into a career in itself. Modeling in France, Germany, and Italy has been the highlight for many young models whose careers started there. (See Chapter 5 under "Making Your Way in Modeling in Other Countries.")

The modeling school is an avenue by which you can glean a little polish, savvy, and a rough idea of the many areas of the work itself. The schools will not let you observe a class in session (as a rule). Therefore you will have to weigh your own abilities and decide whether you feel that you would benefit from this type of school. If you know of someone who has attended a particular school and that person is willing to tell you about it, that might be very helpful.

Fees are commensurate with the area where the school is located, the curriculum, the actual facilities of the school, and the length of the courses taught. There is no guarantee that you will emerge as a model or even that you will get a single job as one.

What might an established modeling school really do for you, and what does it cost?

A school in North Carolina gives modeling, charm classes, pageant preparatory courses, and general self- improvement instruction.

The modeling course includes eight two-hour sessions including:

- posture, carriage, and walk
- diet, exercise, and figure control
- nail care
- skin care
- hair care and styling

- wardrobe coordination and fashion
- etiquette and social graces

The classes are taught by professionals in each field.*

In the advanced modeling course (ten 90-minute sessions), the classes include photographic, runway, stage, and "freeze" modeling; makeup techniques for the stage; and a photography session with a professional photographer who provides the students with a choice of several pictures for their portfolio free of charge. Students completing this course are referred to paid modeling jobs and regularly model in shows put on by the school.

For the Modeling I course, the girls must be thirteen or older. They can take the classes in the daytime or in the evening. The tuition is $90 for the eight two-hour sessions.

A group of classes is also offered for little girls (aged four to eight) at a cost of $25 for two one-hour sessions. The instruction includes modeling, posture, etiquette, and manners. A preteen class for youngsters aged nine to twelve teaches posture, walking, nutrition, exercise, skin and hair care, fashion and color coordination, etiquette, and manners. This six-week course (one hour per week) is $65.

This particular school is located in a rural area where little or no exposure to fashion and self-improvement would otherwise be available. There are occasional fashion shows in the local department store, and students from the school are called upon to model. Some organizations and businesses also provide experience for the students when they organize fashion shows or promotions.

The experience for a prospective model is extremely limited in such an area, but original exposure for many models did not originate in New York or Los Angeles. It is not too difficult to contact neighboring areas and send a

---

*Papillon School of Modeling, flyer. Asheboro, N.C.

letter requesting an interview at one or two of their agencies. Modeling usually pays a high enough wage that it's worth your while to travel a bit for that necessary exposure. You have to be seen to be in demand, and in modeling you have to make every effort to be noticed in the best way possible.

In larger cities, like Atlanta, Cleveland, San Francisco, and Boston, modeling schools are more visible. Some of these schools have associated agencies that help students find work.

If there are more modeling jobs available through these particular school-associated agencies, you may seriously want to look into the school itself, even though you may not feel that you really need the courses. In many middle-sized cities, modeling school classes are more comprehensive, simply due to the demand for more sophisticated modeling work. Thus the tuition is higher. Though it would be impossible to give an exact dollar value from city to city, the average seems to be around $800 for the basics.

A modeling school in New York should be looked into as carefully as any other institution of learning. Merely because it bears a New York City address does not guarantee that it is good. The sessions offered in most New York modeling schools cost between $1200 and about $1500 for the shortest curriculum in all-round modeling. The classes may be spread over as many as nine months or as concentrated as one month. They are for both men and women and should include the basic knowledge needed to start with any agency. Help is given on how to handle your interviews at agencies, what pictures might be needed, and how to compile a resume.

(Remember, if you are planning to go to New York or Los Angeles, that your board and room can be astronomically expensive. You should make concrete inquiries and confirm reservations before your arrival.)

If you are at all fearful of the legitimacy of a school or agency, inquire about it at the Better Business Bureau, an organization that can provide information on the business history and reputation of the school or agency in question.

HAVING PHOTOGRAPHS TAKEN

Only a handful of people can simply step in front of a camera, not feel dreadfully inhibited, and get on with it. Just look through your family album to see those fishy stares while facing that terror—a camera.

An agent once said that after several months, models start to relax enough to be able to present themselves. There is something just dreadfully inhibiting about finding yourself a few feet away from that critical little eye of the camera's lens.

Most photographers try to elicit the right reactions from you with music, subtleties in voice, directions, and atmosphere. Some of the most interesting shoots are taken "on location"—where the product or the fashions would or could most likely be used. Usually, you get to film outside. It's not everybody's idea of fun—the wind, rain, heat, or freezing cold can put a damper on things.

The idea of feeling inhibited must be overcome before you will be able to do your best work in front of the camera. Many agencies in New York who hire you will see to your development. That often means an internship in Europe with many photographers. These photographers will teach you how to move, how to "freeze," how to develop your own special attitude and "look" for the camera. They are known for being very patient and will work with you until they can get the correct "look" on film. The pictures are often quite beautiful, and some are in the various models' books when they return here to continue their careers.

Another way to acquire photographs is to ask other models who did theirs. You can then call the photographer and ask if he or she is testing. If tests are arranged, the model takes the film and pays for processing. The photographer gets to pick from the slides. Both are responsible for their own printing. This benefits both parties, as both need shots for their portfolios. It is a very good way to make contact with as many good photographers as possible. The photographer is often the one who makes recommendations to the client, and that's a plus for you. If you are a good model for the photographer's work, he or she will be able to promote you.

Portfolio

The portfolio is the most important representation of a model and her or his work. Every time you have an appointment for a potential job, you must drop off your portfolio. The client then studies all of the types of photographs that you have displayed and decides whether you would be the perfect model for the work that will be photographed.

Portfolio photographs used to be all 11x14 inch prints, and now many models are using 8½x11s. Check with the agencies of your choice if you are planning on taking professional shots to interviews. Printing is costly and you should think ahead or you may find yourself spending more money than you thought possible.

Most photographs using models are accompanied by the photographer's name, and if you find photographs in a style to your liking, you may want to contact that photographic studio. For television modeling, you have to have photographs going in. The head shots for this specialized type of modeling should depict you at your warmest and friendliest; your fashion work would be unsuitable.

Expect to pay $500 or more for a head shot for television commercials. This would be an 8x10 in black and white that you would have printed, accompanied by your resumé, and leave at all the "possible jobs."

Many times when the selection is to be made, it is only your photograph in a two-foot deep heap of them that reminds the director who was even there. You can see how critical good photographs are to your potential work. There are times also when you may not be selected for the original job that you were seeking and that photograph left on file has been pulled and gotten you another totally unrelated job. One male model was very unhappy about missing out on a particular job, only to have been remembered by the director for his dramatic Japanese good looks. When his photograph was pulled several months later, he was handed not one, but three, really fantastic accounts. His head shot had portrayed him in native Japanese costume while he of course appeared in impeccable western attire for his interview and screen test. The director could see how striking and versatile the model could be. He was just what they were looking for at that future time and my friend had accomplished the greatest hurdle for anyone going on a television audition. Get noticed, and then be the one and only that's remembered. These casting directors see thousands of hopefuls every day and there are many that are pretty much the same, or could feasibly do the same commercial, so they are impressed with the uniqueness that you can project in the two minutes flat that you'll be viewed initially.

EXPENSES AT THE BEGINNING

If you are planning to move to New York or Los Angeles, you will have to have a large nest egg to tide you over, unless you are planning on working at some other job while you try to break into modeling. The rent alone will probably be $400 per month, and that would be sharing a one-bedroom apartment with someone. Many models share their apartments with one or more models. The costs are so high that even studio apartments run $800 per month.

Food will be the next most expensive item in your budget. Food costs in New York City have doubled in the past few years. It used to be possible to save money by cooking at home; now food is so expensive that it is often just as reasonable to go to a neighborhood restaurant. At any rate, your food bill won't be less than $75 per week.

Transportation costs are rising steadily too. New York bus and subway are now 90¢ per ride, and taxis are about $3 a mile in the city.

Medical and dental expenses should be anticipated. You won't be able to fly back to Kansas when your filling comes out in an untimely crunch. A filling could cost about $100. New York is really not a place to be caught without medical insurance coverage.

Add all of the above figures together, plus an allotment for personal items, entertainment, household items, telephone ($100 deposit), and gas and electricity, and you will have an idea of what it could cost you to live in New York.

Add the cost of the photographs that you may initially need, the cost of your portfolio itself ($60), your makeup (which will be extensive if you are a woman), clothing, and any sports gear that you might require. Nobody ever said that New York was an inexpensive city to live in, or that modeling was an inexpensive profession to get into. It is a

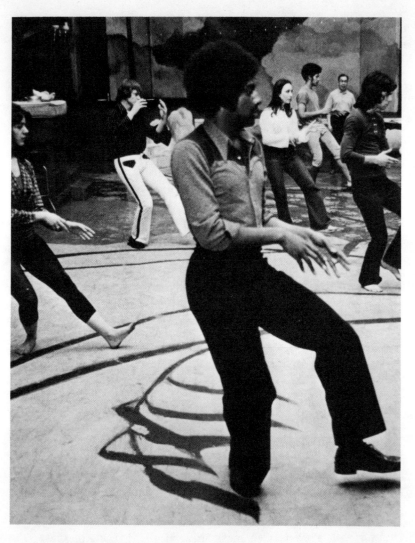

Dance classes will help to develop poise, coordination, grace, and awareness of body positions and balance as well as helping you keep fit. Photo: Columbia College.

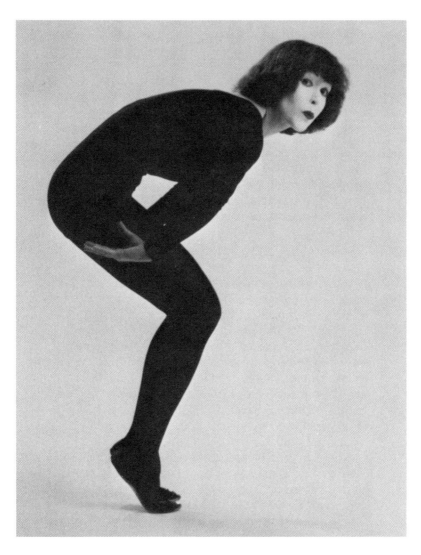

Pantomime and other drama classes will help develop awareness of mood, style, and the ability to communicate feelings. Photo: Chic, Inc.

game to juggle all of the figures; eventually you'll come up with your own solutions on how and where to save pennies.

HELPFUL HINTS

Due to the tremendous competition in the field of modeling, you will want to be as well-prepared prior to your attempted launch into the modeling world as is physically possible. You cannot know exactly what may be the current trend, but you can get yourself in top condition.

Movement

Many agents complain that models who are very good in other areas do not move well enough. There is not only a knack to moving well, but the more trained you are at an early age, the more defined are the long slender muscles that are the trademark of the best-looking people. You must choose carefully what kind of exercise will give those extended lines. Ballet, gymnastics, swimming, and tennis are all very good forms of strenuous exercise and give the body a definitive shape. All of the foregoing are suggested in moderation; three to four hours a week would be ample. You do not want to develop an abundance of muscle.

Wherever your natural forte lies is the best place to put your greatest effort. Many well-known fashion models are simply not graceful to the professional eye, yet they have enough going for them that they are top models. If you watch videos or actual fashion shows, you will see amazing variations in natural grace. Some people move with incredible ease, while others remain visibly uncoordinated throughout their lives.

You can make the *best* of either possible case by starting early to take some kind of regulated exercise and stick with it. A child who starts to take dance lessons before he or she becomes inhibited about moving in front of peers will have a much better chance of overcoming awkwardness. If a child reaches the age of about seven and has never been encouraged to develop any natural abilities like swimming or playing ball, that child may well remain ill-at-ease with any request to move when a possible audience might see her or him.

Teeth

Take excellent care of your teeth! Your smile is a paramount introduction to you—not only for cosmetic reasons, but because bad teeth tell the world that you don't think enough of yourself to take care of them. The male model is primarily noted for his teeth (and his eyes). Men have to have a great smile to sell the product. Women models have to have pretty teeth as part of the whole picture.

Teeth can make or break your career as a model. Many real beauties do not have those perfect teeth and as a result photograph badly. Your teeth could be too far apart, too long, or too irregular. There are many ways to make the needed corrections, and not all of them are even permanent. One famous model uses a spacer between her two front teeth, and only when certain shots require that look. She often models au naturel, with her space between her front teeth as her very own trademark!

Makeup

Makeup is a critical factor for all women models. Applying makeup is an art. When you do a fashion shot, a makeup artist or stylist does your face. This can be as time-consuming as two hours or more. If you are doing catalog and other similar types of work, you will have to do your own makeup, and well.

There are many tricks of the trade. Some of these can be picked up at places where makeup artists work on you, advise you as they go along, and show you how to bring out your best features. You are expected to buy makeup, but you also will pay for the makeup artists' work. Shading and highlighting are two of the most important things that you have to learn.

To do your makeup really well, you must understand what the camera sees and try to correct any flaws that nature has given you. If you have circles under the eyes, for example, you will want to use a small amount of moisturizer and cover it lightly with powder. This is a hard area to disguise and the less done the better. As you get older, less and less makeup is used. Heavy makeup only attracts the eye to the deepened facial lines, and the camera is very quick to pick up on all the imperfections accented by bad makeup.

In using makeup, you will discover the difference between what is worn in front of the camera versus what is worn in natural light. There are many tricks that involve shading. Dark colors make the object recede or seem less prominent, while light colors bring the object forward.

Lips, cheeks, and noses are all treated in special ways to make the best possible presentation. It will take you a while to gain the knack of how to handle all those makeup brushes, bottles, blends, cakes, pastes, and wands, but time will make you adept. Eventually you will be confident with your own ability to make your face look its best.

Fingernails

Your fingernails don't always need to be painted, but they have to be perfectly manicured. That means they should be really scrubbed, with no visible cuticle, and either coated with clear polish or buffed to a soft shine. Your nails are right out there, and there is no way to hide a lack of care on your part. Become adept with the emery board, and be able to keep both hands looking neat. Once you've started to make an income as a model, you'll want to head straight to the manicurist and the pedicurist once a week. The pedicurist will do to your feet what the manicurist does to your hands. These services cost about $30 plus tip.

Legs

Leg waxing is critical for a model and is done on an as-you-need-it basis. Most women go to the salon at least once every six weeks, but if you are averse to all this time-consumption you may desire removal of hair from bikini line, legs, mustache, underarms, and eyebrows by electrolysis. In the long run it could save you money and time.

Fashion Sense

Try to develop your fashion sense as soon as possible. Exposure to art classes, sewing courses, and familiarization with costume in museums and libraries are all helpful. You are not normally expected to create any of your ensembles for actual modeling work, but your own fashion sense will be valuable in your presentation of the clothing in front of the camera, and in your presentation of yourself.

If you are paid to be a model, you are expected to look

like one. That doesn't mean loads of makeup and thousand dollar ensembles, but it does mean clean, neat, and a certain amount of care given to your appearance. You never know whom you may meet, and a model has to be an opportunist. Often a job is offered when you least expect it. Not all jobs are found through go-sees. You are your own best advertisement, and the sooner you prepare yourself for self-sell, the better. So much of modeling is based on merely your looks that the best presentation possible won't hurt you either!

Performance

Acting lessons, speech lessons, and voice instruction may be very helpful if you are aiming toward television work as part of your modeling profession. Any plays having a possible part for you should be given serious preparation and an audition.

Every experience that you could possibly have before an audience—choral singing, plays, variety shows, beauty pageants, and even attending social functions—can be helpful in giving you that critical self-confidence. Poise is gained by experience. Though modeling can only be done *well* by the truly experienced *model*, your efforts to meet the public and feel at ease in front of lots of people can aid you tremendously when you are asked to "perform" before the cameras.

If you wait until you are actually offered an audition for a television part to start to learn to speak well and dramatize a little, you probably will freeze, and lose the part.

Many soap opera stars started as models and now enjoy much more financial security because they added the important talent of speech to their repertory of mime while they were still photographic models. Being prepared and being lucky enough to be there at the right time are the magical combination.

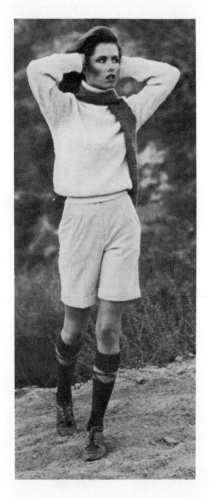 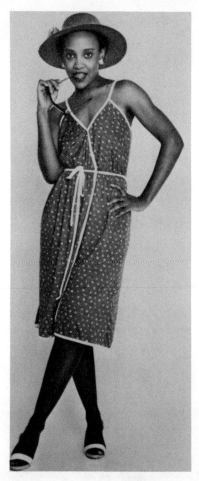

Some of the best money is to be made in fashion work. Photos: Chic, Inc.

CHAPTER 5

WHAT CAN YOU EXPECT TO EARN?

Full-time modeling in New York or Los Angeles, the two capitals of fashion in the United States, could reward you with a salary in the millions if you are one of the very successful high fashion models. Obviously, there are not too many people that far up the ladder, so we'll start on the bottom rung and give you an idea of what kind of money is out there, where the big money is being made, and how to organize your career in the direction of a substantial salary for yourself.

MODELING OUTSIDE AND INSIDE OF NEW YORK OR LOS ANGELES

In a small city, you would primarily draw a salary for live promotional work. This work is most often paid at approximately double the minimum wage. Promotional models are usually hired for the hours of ten to four, as the public to whom the products are usually presented are in the stores during those hours.

Runway work is usually paid at $25 per hour and could run a bit more or less depending on the time of year, the actual promoters, the number of models needed, and the size of the return expected from that showing. If the show is a very lavish one and for an extended length of time, that will be taken into consideration and the pay could run as high as about $50 per hour. Runway and fashion shows do not always have cash remuneration in the smaller cities, however, and pay may be made in clothing or even in makeup.

There are also photographic jobs available in moderation, depending on the size of the city and how prominent it is in the local fashion world. For the department store's advertising in the local newspapers and brochures, you could expect to be paid about $50 per hour.

Agencies in rural areas have a set rate for which the model may be hired. That rate would apply to whatever job the model might be requested to do, from live promotional work (where he or she might otherwise only make the doubled minimum wage) to photographic work. The agency and thus the model might be paid $25 per hour, for example. This seems quite fair in that the agency then looks for better-paying jobs and you have a chance at developing a reasonable income. The idea here is that you would like to be a model *only* and not have to subsidize your income forever with other work.

Local manufacturers sometimes hire models for their showrooms. Such work though seasonal pays about $15 to $20 per hour. The work is only available a few weeks during the year, so you could not consider making a living from it.

In a middle-sized city where a model works at all of the aforementioned, there is simply not enough income available from modeling for you to have a real career of it. Ultimately, to make a career in modeling, you have to move to Chicago, Dallas, New York, or Los Angeles. The experience gleaned in a smaller town will have given you a bit of self-confidence and will hold you in good stead. You will learn that having done your homework in any sized city is what forms the basis of professionalism.

The high fashion industry is the only place where you can make a really full-time career as a model and be financially independent. This is true for both men and women. Though the male model could never hope to compete with a high fashion model in salary or career, he could certainly make a sizable income in the fashion capitals.

Not long ago the top salaries for the fashion models in the middle- sized cities ranged from $6000 to $10,000 a year. These were the best and the busiest models, and yet that was all the work that was available to them. Women in New York City who are just starting out with an agency are paid between $75 and $300 per hour depending on the kind of modeling. Male models in New York City have starting pay of between $75 and $175 per hour depending on the agency. Some will and do pay up to the $300 per hour.

The way to build up your hourly wage is by building up your notoriety. The agency pushes their top models; if you work your way up to that category, you could be making the over-$100,000 salary. A particular look comes in, and if you are that look, you'll have to capitalize upon it quickly. Fashion can be quite fickle. While you are the in look, you will have to move fast.

Catalog Work

There are many areas in which you could start reaping in these salaries. The first area is known for its bread-and-butter support of models—catalog work. You've seen hundreds of catalogs stuffing your mailbox, especially around Christmas time. The catalogs are distributed from department stores, mail order houses, food importers, sporting

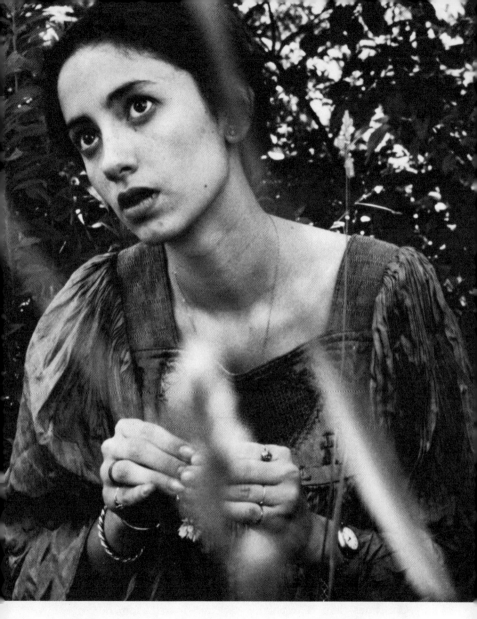

Fees paid for certain unusual mood and location shots will range widely. Photo: SWG.

goods merchandisers, toy manufacturers, travel packagers, and many more. The companies hire models to demonstrate their wares or beam unself-consciously in everything from silk underwear to million dollar furs and diamond necklaces. The more prestigious items will be modeled by the highest paid models. Though the salary may start at $75 to $150 per hour in the bigger agencies, your potential is really unlimited, and there are catalog jobs that are extremely well paid. If a model's fee is $500 per hour, and a client has that look in mind as the marketable face, that client knows what prestige a known model's face can bring to the product and its sales. It is becoming very popular to have a known face and figure rather than an unknown—thus the constant search for new models who could become the coveted look of tomorrow. There is a similarity in the look of many of the known models and though there is a professed trend to deviate from the tall-blonde-and-leggy, the demand from the clients still keeps them the highest on the demand list.

The *editorial rate* for the high fashion models is generally pretty low. The current rate is around $90 per day starting pay. Editorial is the work that is print but not commercial like the actual promotion of a product such as soap or toothpaste. A model must do this kind of work in combination with commercial catalog work to survive. Generally speaking, any woman in high fashion could do catalog work but many of the models that you see doing work in catalogs are not high fashion models. For catalog work, you generally do your own makeup; for fashion work, it is usually done for you.

You can tell by looking at the models if they are high fashion or not. Doing so should be part of your preparation for a modeling career. Scan the material that comes your way for the qualities of the fashion model. Your eye will become accustomed to a certain polished "look" and demeanor. You won't be able to distinguish this by what they are promoting or what they are wearing, but by the stance, projection of attitude, and "feel" of the model.

The more projection the model has the better the "look" of that person will be remembered, and that's what will make the hourly rate skyrocket.

You will want to do a mixture of both catalog work and fashion work. Without catalog work, you will have no money as the pay scale is good ($75-$100) per hour, but without fashion work you won't hold your own in the industry. So you must have a good balance of these two types of work to remain a photographic model represented by an agency.

You are of course paid for your time while you are being made up, having your hair styled and having the clothing fitted before a photographic session.

Runway Work and Fashion Shows

There are some high-paying and some rather moderate rates for the same type of work. Runway work that is done in various hotels for business groups and some social functions are occasionally done by models just starting in the field, some fresh out of a modeling school. The models are offered this experience in exchange for photographs and are not remunerated in cash. The photographs and the experience itself are both very valuable to the inexperienced model.

Informal modeling in department stores in New York is on a pay scale of about $75 per hour. These are the models who do the fashion work in everything from expensive gowns to bathing suits in the largest stores. They are always exceedingly thin but not necessarily photogenic.

Big fashion shows could pay as little as $100 to $150 per hour. The model is compensated at half that pay while being fitted. The fees can go much higher than the aforementioned rates. One Seventh Avenue showroom pays $250 per hour for runway work. Depending on where it is in the world and where the show lies in the fashion season, more or less will be paid.

If you choose to work for a showroom on Seventh Avenue as a model, you will gain experience but not get paid a great deal. This is a weekly job with a weekly salary. Some models like the security of the nine-to-five job, but the difference in your potential salary is significant. The weekly salary would vary according to your experience and the type of garments that you are required to wear.

Much of Seventh Avenue does not require a high fashion model, and there is work to be found there even if you are as short as five feet, six inches. You need only be moderately attractive and pleasant in personality, as you deal directly with customers. You could be modeling any garment from junior sportswear to bathing suits. Current weekly salaries for the huge variety of Seventh Avenue models can be found in the want ads in the local papers. Pay in the smaller department stores is currently about $45 per hour.

Go to several interviews if you plan to work on Seventh Avenue or the department stores. It will give you an idea where you will fit in best. Both are live modeling jobs and both could potentially lead to other things. The main difference is the figure types required. The Seventh Avenue model *could* be the shorter, bustier girl. The department store model who shows women's clothing will have to be at least five feet, eight inches or taller and less than 120 pounds. Some Seventh Avenue models will have the high fashion prerequisites also. If this seems a bit confusing, it is because the garment district has very different needs in their models than high fashion alone.

All you would have to do to get a clearer idea of who might be modeling on Seventh Avenue is to wander through the endless sections of junior to large-size clothing in the stores. If a garment is sold, it potentially was modeled for a buyer at some point. The way to narrow the field is to read the specifications in the daily want ads that are calling for models for the garment section.

A whole new group of models, women over five feet, eight inches tall and weighing 150 to 200 pounds, have recently come into demand. Such women are needed by the market to model the clothing that a vast number of women now need. Not only are more women taller than they ever were, but they are proportionately filled out. These models can find work not only on Seventh Avenue, but also in photographic work to sell the large-size clothing. The salary level here is one of more than $100,000, potentially, per year. Everything from large-sized swimming suits to evening gowns needs to be modeled, so there are plenty of jobs available in this area. Not all agencies handle the large-size model, but you would definitely want to be handled by an agency to guarantee the highest income, unless you wanted to start in the garment district where you would be a weekly salaried employee.

A good model who has just started out should not expect to make anything for the first three months. After that, the jobs should start coming in and the model should reasonably expect to have at least three jobs a week. By the beginning of the second year, you should be making at least $50,000 and from then on the sky is the limit. You will bring in just as much as you yourself are willing to work for. There are always appointments to go to. If you are enthusiastic and have the needed look, you'll be out there perhaps six or seven times every day on "go-sees." No one who has ever worked as a model could ever call it anything but very hard work!

The model who pushes constantly could certainly see the salary above $100,000.

You will want to do jobs with as much variety as possible to take advantage of your youth. Remember that this job as a career cannot last past the age of twenty-three, unless you are extremely lucky and your face shows no lines. So you have to work extra hard every day, make absolutely certain that you really want this so badly that you're willing to give your all, and you're sure to make it!

With a good agency behind you, and the two of you cooperating on your career, you might just become one of the million dollar models! You'll never know unless you get out there and explore the field. You have to start early. Right now is not too soon!

MAKING YOUR WAY IN MODELING IN OTHER COUNTRIES

Modeling in Europe as a way of entering the field is becoming more and more popular. When you are signed by an agency, an apprenticeship (period of learning) in Europe to work with fashion, makeup, photographers, and how to handle yourself and paraphernalia usually lasts about six months. At that time, most fashion models return to their agencies in the United States. If you should be lucky enough to land some paying work in Europe, you could find yourself working in England, Sweden, Denmark, Belgium, France, Holland, Germany, or Italy. If you decide to return to any of these countries at a later time, you will probably find enough modeling work to keep you happy and enjoy Europe as well.

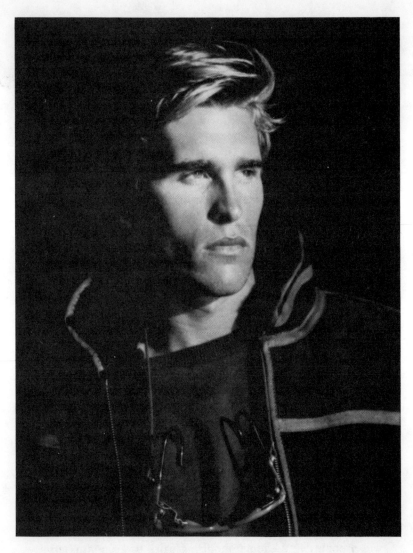

Carey Stokes' pleasantly rugged looks make him well suited for outdoor and sports work. Photo: Ford Men, by Pieter Estersohn.

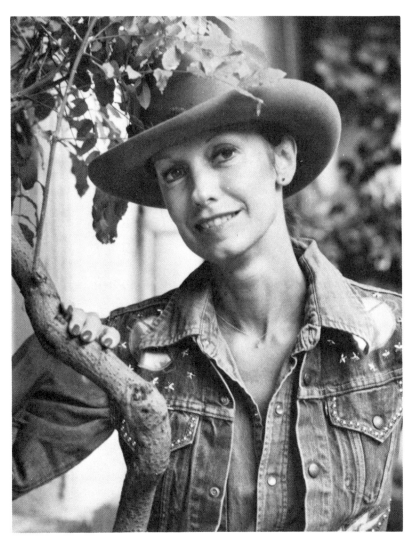

The author, on freelance assignment. Photo: SWG.

There are of course many "on location" jobs where an American model or several models are sent to work. These stays are not lengthy, and many models complain that they have been places but had so little time to sightsee that they don't know anything about where they were. At some point in your career, you may want to relocate. The money to be made in modeling is excellent worldwide.

The Japanese market is opening ever wider to the Western models. Many young blonde models have been there this past year and really raved about their experiences. Many catalogs and brochures have featured American models in China, in just the past few years. Most American models who have relocated for any length of time live in Europe.

EXCLUSIVE CONTRACT FOR A PRODUCT

Many models hope for an exclusive contract with a company whose product they are hired to represent in every type of media possible. The people who first come to mind are those women whose faces have been the sole (or almost the only one) model for the huge cosmetic companies. What exclusivity means is that the model will only be photographed in that company's cosmetics. This prohibiting act (on the part of the company) is very expensive for the client. By cutting off the model's other possible sources, the hiring company contracts her at a fee that must satisfy her and compensate for all the other potential work that she might have been able to do. Exclusivity is so very highly paid that most models are very desirous of such an arrangement. The best part of this type of contract is of course the security and the fame that comes with being associated with some of the most prestigious products.

Exclusivity contracts have been known to go over $200,000 per year, and every year these plum jobs get even higher dollar fees.

INEXPERIENCED VERSUS
EXPERIENCED MODELS' FEES

The fees indicated in this chapter for the various types of modeling are all the bottom rates. As a model becomes more well known, and more in demand, the agency will raise her or his fee. It works somewhat like the supply and demand in any business. The model's fees keep increasing and level off when the demand does. The demand could just stop altogether too, so one has to be prepared for many eventualities.

Always be prepared for the best *and* the worst. No one can predict the future. Some of the women and men who looked like they were going to set the world on fire, within a month fizzled almost instantaneously.

Experienced models' fees, if all goes well, are often over $100,000 per year.

The lucky and very rare model whose career takes flight instantaneously could make that half million dollar salary or more! Only one model in hundreds of thousands will make it at all, and the ratio of becoming a super model is much greater than even that.

The models who are making such high yearly salaries are combining many forms of modeling—high fashion, runway, television, catalog, editorial work, videos, and even posters. The money to be made from all of these sources collectively is stupifying!

While the model is a look that is salable, the money must be made and quickly. Youth does not wait, and popularity can and does wane, so the clever model makes all the money possible during the halcyon days.

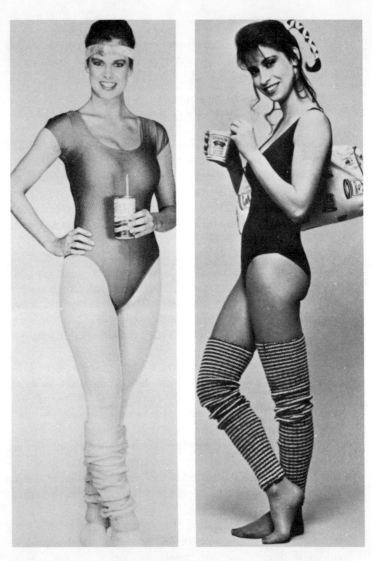

You may choose an agency based on the kind of work you want to do and are best suited for. Photos: Chic, Inc.

CHAPTER 6

THE MODELING AGENCY

There are hundreds of agencies in New York City alone that represent models. When you set out to find the right agency to represent you, keep these things in mind. *After* you have signed a contract with an agency it will be too late to reconsider what you should have been looking for.

CHOOSING A MODELING AGENCY

It is up to you to choose the agency that you think could use your particular "look" to the optimum. Every agency specializes in a certain style. Familiarize yourself with the various models that each agency represents. You will see the similarities in their overall look, and you must then judge where you think that you fit in best.

Weigh the advantages and the disadvantages of the smaller versus the larger agency prior to calling for an appointment. A smaller agency would more than likely be able to get you more work, but their pay scale could be as low as half of what you could make at one of the bigger agencies! One tremendous advantage to working for a smaller agency is that if you are completely green, you will gain experience and become polished in the interim.

The bigger agency is in a better position to pay the larger fees to models. Your pay scale could be doubled with a large agency, but you could also find yourself working less as the calls would be spread more thinly amongst the many models. Though you may be being sent on nearly twice the number of go-sees as the smaller agency could send you on, the larger agency has more models for that same client to interview for the same job.

After you have made an appointment for an interview at the agency of your choosing, you will start the process of what you hope will be the perfect match.

At that all-important interview, let them do the talking. Listen carefully and answer all of their questions as concisely as you can. Most of the questions will be to establish your height and measurements and to get a reasonable understanding of what you expect from the modeling world and how you think that the agency will fit into the scheme of things.

Questions like "Why do you want to model?" and "Why do you think that you would be good at it?", are just a few of the things they'll be likely to ask. Remember that they can be very personal and be prepared to take this likelihood in stride.

At your interview, do not be modest, but do not brag either. Any extra talent that the agency may be able to promote for you is money in your pocket and theirs. If you are a good athlete, dancer, skin diver, or even were in many serious dramatic productions, be sure to mention it at your interview. There are many occasions where a model is required to show off ski gear, and it may not be from a chair-lift alone! Don't exaggerate when it comes to your actual ability. You may get caught in your own web, and find yourself at the top of the hill with all the cameras on you *waiting* for you to actually ski down!

No one can tell you beforehand if you will be hired by any agency; on the other hand you may be offered a contract within minutes of your interview. Be prepared for both possibilities. You cannot take the lack of an offer as a personal rejection, as the interviewer may honestly believe that you might fit in better somewhere else, in which case to hire you would be a disservice to both of you. If an interviewer sees no future in creating a business relationship, you must take it as a positive statement and simply look into another agency. It is less likely that you will have to go to more than one interview if you genuinely try to understand *who* are the types of models that each agency represents. One very pretty young woman worked in an agency for a few months; having been employed in their office, she then set out to try the modeling end of things. She got up her courage, sized up all of the agencies, selected the one she thought best for her, and she was hired on the spot. Working on the inside for a summer gave her the discerning judgement to know where she fit into an agency.

Having been just hired by an agency, you cannot even imagine how much that agency can guide your destiny. It is up to them to send you where you can potentially perform at your very best for both of you. You are in business together and though they may be able to open some doors, your own caliber of work and self-sell will have to keep those doors open.

An agency will sign you only if they feel that the contract will be mutually beneficial. This means that the agency will do everything in their power to promote you, to get auditions and interviews lined up for you, and to make you into a more salable look. Therefore, it is of paramount importance that you and your agency are not only compatible, but really honest and straightforward with one another.

Fees

The agency must set your fees wisely for the various types of work that they and you expect to be doing. The agency will set up your go-sees and it is up to you to give it all you've got—to get to the appointment on time looking great, make the right impression, and present your book and yourself as professionally as possible.

The agency is there to protect you. Once they have set your fees and you have done a job, the agency will bill the client and collect your fee. You are responsible to your agency for a percentage of your fee as theirs for services rendered. There are no set percentages, but you can expect to have your agent charge between 15 and 20 per cent. That seems to be the most common, but there are agencies that charge more. Be certain that these things are spelled out clearly in your contract.

THE AGENT'S JOB

The agency is your answering service, business manager, bookkeeper, secretary, advisor, tutor, and even your guide as to weight reduction, hair styles, makeup, and diet.

The agency protects you from unscrupulous clients and unprofessional people with whom you may come in contact. A model does not have to accept a particular job if he or she does not wish to. The power of the agency can make it very difficult for less than legitimate contacts.

The agency sees to the right model selection for go-sees. It is their business to comprehend what the client wants, and that model will be dispatched. It behooves the agency to have very clever people in its employ for discretionary selection. If they judge incorrectly, a model from another agent gets the job.

When the agency sets up the go-see, the model is always advised as to what to take to the particular appointment. Frequently the garment to be worn is see-through or nearly so, and one wise model says that she never goes anywhere without bringing a bra as she's found them required many times when the agency would never have thought of it.

Once under contract, you have actually to be sent on many go-sees to get started. If you are working in a small, slower agency, you could see three to four clients a day. A larger agency might send you on as many as seven or eight go-sees a day.

You will only have a few months; then if you do not start to "move," the agency may lose interest in you. Those first weeks are the make or break probationary time, so you have to convey your uniqueness, charm, and effervescence in a hurry.

If you are planning to move to a large city to work for an agency, they will often help you find housing. Ask your agent about this possibility if you are going to have to relocate to work for their agency.

Agencies are divided into different divisions if they handle large numbers of men, women, children, and a variety of television, runway work, and shows. There is so much complex work involved that it would be next to impossible to cope with the needs intelligently without having the various sections. Many models take advantage of as many kinds of work as their agency can offer them.

Many models feel that you are not taken as seriously if you try to freelance (work without being represented by any agent). A city like New York is so big that unless you have many personal contacts and know all the ropes, you are likely to find it nearly impossible to operate as a freelance model. The major benefit to being a freelance model is that you would not have any agency fees to consider into your budget. But if you cannot *get* any modeling jobs without the aid of the agents, then of course you have saved half of nothing.

Composites

Most big agencies help defray expenses in that they will pay for your composites. These are rather small cards with several photographs of you arranged in some sort of fashionable array. The composite is made of several of your selected photographs and is left as your calling card at the clients' when you have completed a go-see. This little card often gets you work at some future date, as the client can then open a file, and though you may not have been perfect for the original job, you may be for subsequent ones.

Portfolios

Portfolios can be dreadfully expensive, and the book itself could cost $600. One print could easily run $10 to $20, and you'll need at least 10 to 12 different prints. By the time that you will have completed a good portfolio, it will have cost about $1000. However a good agency will help you build up your portfolio by "testing" (they send you to the photographers and in return you and the photographer will each have prints) and spare you the cost of paying for the best photographers.

Your portfolio is extremely important. It is your most necessary tool of the trade. The clients must see how you look in print. The photographs in your book should give the widest range possible of your "looks" and allow the clients to have some insight into *how* you potentially will look in their commercial or print ad.

The agency should also help you to select the photographs that are the best ones for your portfolio. Their keen eye for what is good is honed through many years in the business, and their experience is valuable to both you and them financially.

Control

An agency has a great deal of control over whom you will or won't work with through their selection of the models sent on go-sees. A good agency behind you can literally make you, as opportunities are made available for you to work your way up the ladder. The agent sets up the critical connections, and you have to cement them. With a large amount of luck, pluck, and energy, you can make it in the modeling field. The hardest part is getting started. Now that you know that the agency has put its vote of confidence in you, the rest is up to you!

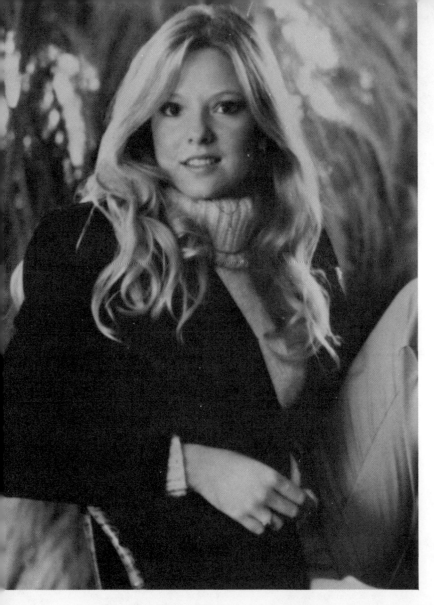

The advantages of a modeling career may include interesting assignments, pleasant contacts, and variety of work. Photo: Chic, Inc.

CHAPTER 7

ADVANTAGES AND DISADVANTAGES OF BEING A MODEL

What one person does with ease and grace just may be another's nemesis. So as you read the following lists of advantages and disadvantages, keep in mind that these were either personally experienced or related by various models who have worked in the many fields of modeling.

ADVANTAGES ACCORDING TO THE MODELS

- "The money is terrific. Nobody would *think* of paying me the kind of money that I make as a model, so I plan to stick with it as long as I can."
- "The best part is getting to go 'on location' because it's usually somewhere pretty exotic, and it was out of the question that I'd ever get to see any of these places before I got to be a model. I've been to Italy, Japan, and Greece is a possibility."
- "Just having been a model for as long as I have been was an experience that no one could take away from me. It was a kind of an education in itself."
- "It does have a lot of prestige in certain circles, and the contacts are great."

- "Some people think that it's a pretty glamourous job, and I agree with them! My lifestyle is so different now."
- "I love wearing all the beautiful and some pretty weird things too. It's theater on its own level."
- "I just happened to be lucky. My girlfriend and I started out together, and even though she is really a beauty naturally, I'm the bigger success because I wanted it so much more."
- "You get a lot of self-confidence from working as a model. Between the rejection and the praise it can be a little much, but it keeps you going if your head is where it should be. I know that I'm a good model, and that it's hard work. It gives me self-satisfaction."

DISADVANTAGES ACCORDING TO THE MODELS

- "You always have to promote yourself. Your agency sends you out on a go-see and the rest is up to you."
- "You always have to be 'up' and even after days of being told that you're not the person for that particular job, you *can't* let yourself feel dejected. It's all part of the game."
- "You never know how long a client will want you to represent the product. It's a real day-to-day risk."
- "I never can eat whatever I'd like. I have to think of the deprivation tomorrow if I have pizza tonight."
- "The hardest thing is that I can't go out to parties. I really have to be in bed early, and it really shows up on the camera if you haven't had at least eight to nine hours of sleep."
- "I'm really torn between continuing my modeling and getting a degree that I know I'll need very soon. The

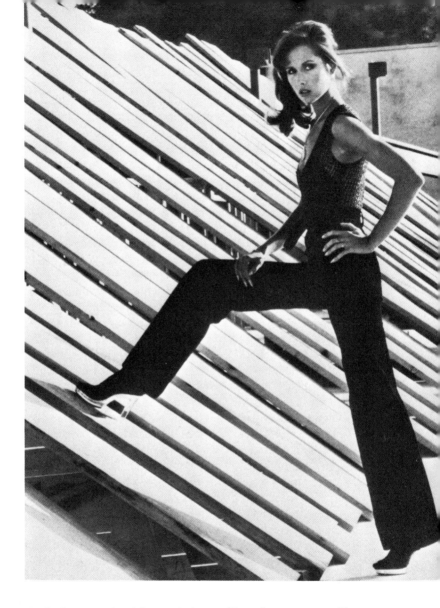

The disadvantages of modeling may be long or tiring assignments, competition for jobs, and the ebb and flow of availability of work. Photo: Chic, Inc.

money is great right now, but I'll have to be behind all my friends if I put off my college until later.''

- ''It's hard to be in a profession where you know that you'll be a *has-been* by the time you're 22.''
- ''It really is extremely hard work, and everyone who's never modeled somehow thinks that the end result was gotten by my standing around looking pretty.''
- ''I think that I really miss my sense of privacy most. That is the price you pay for notoriety.''
- ''You just have to be there at the right time. It's been really frustrating!''
- ''The stress is incredible! I feel guilty if I'm tired.''
- ''Go-sees are really nerve-wracking. It would be great to get all of your work through recommendation.''
- ''New York is a hard market to crack. You have to be a strong person. It's a vicious business, and you have to sift through it. You have to see it for what it is.''
- ''You have to provide your clothing. They do not give you the clothes that you model. That's just not true.''
- ''The fact that you never know that you will definitely have work worries me. I want to know that I'll be able to meet my bills. So many of us are out there now.''
- ''It's the kind of work where you just don't meet anyone to date. My hours and the fact that I work with mostly women can make life a little lonely.''
- ''The worst part for me is seeing how great the more seasoned models' books are. It'll take me a long time to get my photographs up there.''
- ''The discipline is really rigid. I wish that I could take a break from my diet, exercise program and daily schedule, but if I'm not visible, there are just so many other girls who are dying for the work that I can't relax!''
- ''My boyfriend accuses me of being self-centered. I

know that modeling is a 24-hour job, and if I don't watch out for my future jobs, nobody else will. We fight a lot about how much time my work takes me away from our relationship, but I really want to model, and I hope that we can stay together too.''

- ''Sometimes the jobs are really boring. I try to pretend that they aren't by thinking of other things, but you have to keep your mind on what's going on so that you're responsive. It's only good when you're getting a variety of work, and that doesn't always happen.''
- ''I find that New York is so unhealthy compared to my native state, and I would give anything to be able to have my career in modeling back in the Mid-West. I know that's just impossible, but I'll stick it out here for a while longer because the money is so unbelievable.''
- ''It's hard to put up with some of the temperaments of the designers, stylists, and even some of the other models, but personality conflicts can be a problem in any line of work.''

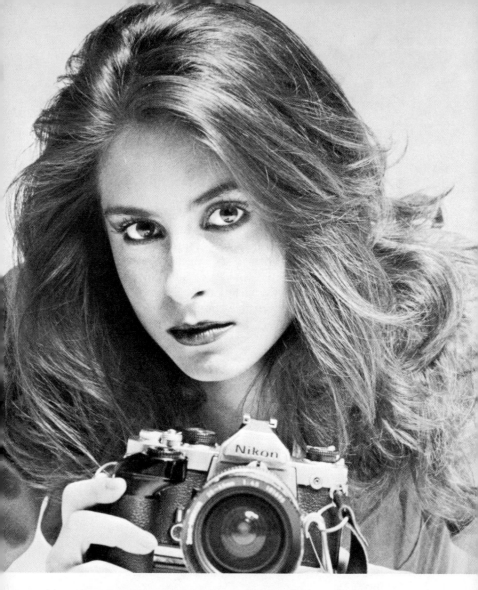

Related careers may include writing, photography, design, or costuming, among others. Photo: Michelle Sereen of Chic, Inc., by John Warner.

CHAPTER 8

AFTER MODELING IS FINISHED

No models should be so unprepared for the end of their modeling life that they have not given it serious thought. If you have made huge amounts through the years of your modeling career and have a cache somewhere, you may not even have to face the (financial) future for many years to come.

If you are a woman, the "plan-ahead" time should be every week that you are working as a model. Time has a way of escaping, and even if you are only in your teens, your modeling career *could* be over before you reach 20—if your "look" stops moving.

Be prepared for the eventuality, and if it doesn't come for many years, then you can just keep making your nest egg bigger and bigger.

You may work as a model only for several months, or maybe not that long. So save some of your money for a transition to your next line of work.

There are many model-related fields that can and do offer work that is sometimes an offshoot of your actual work in front of the camera like continuing to work with models with *you* as the organizer or agent.

RELATED WORK

The type of work sought by models most frequently, when their modeling careers are waning is in the field of *acting*. This a natural sort of extension, in that you are still working in front of cameras, still being the ham. The major difference is you have to have or develop acting ability. Many models have tried this route only to discover that they fizzled as actors and actresses. Others are still out there in the public eye doing everything from videos to full-fledged Hollywood movies. They were smart enough to use modeling as a steppingstone and made the connections needed while they were models. Television commercials prepared many of them with the knowledge of how to handle auditions and with the self-confidence and experience needed to cross over into movies.

Movie starlettes are rarely acting wizards. Most of them are extremely attractive, so with a little luck the acting ability can be perfected on the way up. It is paramount that you photograph well, and you have that under your belt from the modeling experience. If you were or are a successful model, your chances of getting a part in a film are reasonable.

You have to follow your own desires when you are seeking another job. Though movies, television- or Hollywood-style are in the offing, don't just take them because someone *else* thinks that they are a terrific career. There are many types of work that you could do happily and well, so look around.

PHOTOGRAPHY

If you really are enthralled with fashion, there are many possibilities in conjunction with this area. Some models have made excellent *photographers*, because they understand something of the work after years in front of the lens. The creativity in this field has been fascinating to many models. A wide field of work could come from your endeavors.

Photography is very competitive and pretty much a self-sell occupation, much like modeling. The income to be made from this profession would depend on your choice of location, but if you pick a fashion center like New York or Los Angeles, you could expect to start at $20,000. Good fashion photographers make salaries many many times that on an annual basis.

You may want to apprentice yourself to a photographer for a while and learn all of the inside tricks of the trade. As an assistant you won't make much money, but it may be the best way to enter the field.

There are several other areas of work that are involved with the photographic world, from stylist to makeup artist.

The *stylist* is responsible for the "look" to be created on the model. The hair, clothing, makeup, mood, and composite of the entire picture falls to the stylist. A real fashion sense comes into play here. You would put all of your past experience to work and be creative as well.

FASHION WORK

Fashion coordinators do work for department stores, fashion shows, and the like. Their work entails putting together clothing ensembles from shoes upward. There are many ensembles put together by fashion coordinators that are eventually the way the outfits become worn on the street or as a special costume.

Fashion designers are another whole group of fashion-conscious men and women—the core of the business. The designers create the look, and the model and the press carry it to the outside world. Fashion design entails an awareness of art, pattern-making, the ability to sew (enough to understand *how* the pattern is going to fit), color coordination, marketing, and promotion.

This is a pretty tough field to tackle, but you may really love the area. In that case you will need schooling at a fashion institute, and a great deal of luck. This is a very competitive and over-crowded field. Many start in it, and many more drop out due to the talented people already in the field.

If you have any writing talent, you may want to go into the editorial end of fashion. *Beauty editors* are often women who were or could have been fashion models, and who have that sixth sense of what makes fashion and how to describe it to the public. Many fashions are presented to the world on the written page. These are not only exciting but also key jobs in the fashion world.

Some Seventh Avenue fashion models go directly into the *retail business*, as the work that they are involved in often includes sales. There are commissions to be made in this area, and if you are adept at sales, you may want to consider retail. Sales is the area that is currently opening to women at the fastest pace. There are several ways that you could stay in the fashion world with retail work.

Promotion and sales of every possible product in the fashion world could be handled by women. They understand the product and are excellent at the sales end of it. One of the biggest markets outside of the clothing industry is the makeup industry. This is another huge area in which women excel. Many directors of beauty and fashion are women, and some are former fashion models. Who could be more qualified than a beautiful woman who understands what women aspire to be?

When a fashion model leaves her chosen field of modeling at an age somewhere in her early twenties, she is at the prime point in her life to take responsibility for a decision-making job. She certainly will have had much experience in discipline, self-sell, fashion awareness, competition, and a healthy dose of maturity. All of these traits are tremendous assets for the beauty industry to utilize. The wisdom of what makes fashion and beauty is the ongoing interest of the field. The women and men who were involved in one area of the fashion job market have often circulated to other areas and enriched all the facets of fashion in so doing.

Fashion illustrators are another critical group in the fashion world. As a model you may have sat for these artists. Their contribution is one of the stylized trademarks of the printed fashion world. Their work can be viewed everywhere, from museums to the daily newspapers. This is a very competitive field, one that employs a fine art.

Art school and a good bit of natural talent are the criteria. Some models have made it in this field, as some of them started out as illustrators and switched to modeling while the chance was offered. The four-year fashion school is the usual channel for entering fashion illustration; that schooling could run concurrently with your modeling career.

As the third largest industry in the United States, the fashion business has myriad job possibilities, and you'll want to put this foremost in your mind during your modeling career. The contacts that you make while you are modeling could be extremely helpful in your pursuit of future areas of work. Keep the contacts in mind, and keep their business cards as references in case you are interested in that particular area of work.

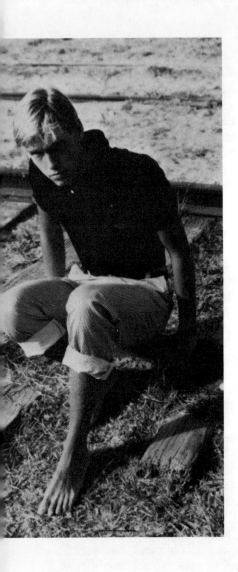

Male models may do casuals, sportswear, business and formal wear. Photos: above, James Mischka. Below, Pivot Point.

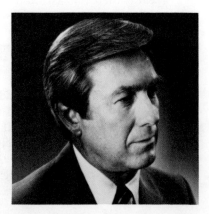

CAREER SPAN FOR MEN

For male models, the decision will not be so critical. Male models who are successful can continue to work long into their late-middle years if they so desire. There are male models who have never had to seek another type of work and have lived well on their modeling incomes their entire adult lives. The fact that many major modeling agencies have expanded to accommodate male model divisions testifies to the fact that the men are really making their own mark in a once totally female-dominated world.

Male models who want to leave the field of modeling for various reasons (not the least of which could be lack of work) could easily fit into the sales end of fashions. Their fashion awareness would hold them in good stead, and the money to be made is substantial. Many men go into design from modeling work as they have learned *what* is needed and desirable to the market. Many innovative styles are model-initiated. Much of the fashion world overlaps and it is not surprising to see the needs of one area fulfilled by the intuitiveness of another.

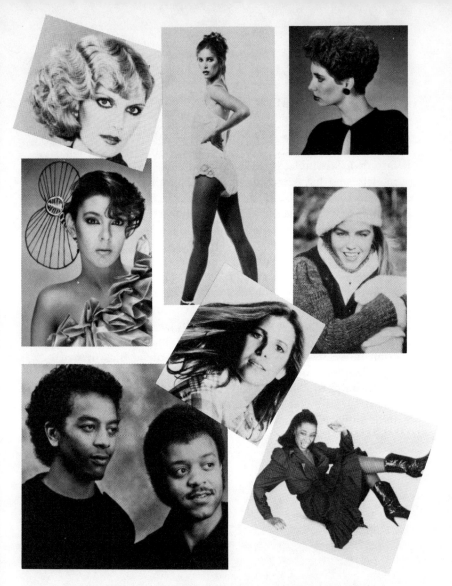

A good range of models will be needed to start an agency. Photos: Upper left, left center, lower left, and upper right, Pivot Point; top center, center, right center, and lower right, Chic, Inc.

CHAPTER 9

OWNING YOUR OWN MODELING AGENCY OR MODELING SCHOOL

After working for several years as a model, you feel that you know the business inside and out. You may want to take on another related or even unrelated type of work. You may want to have your own agency to handle models and guide them on their way toward a career.

Many years ago, an enterprising woman saw the need for organizing the many facets of promotional modeling done within the various department stores in New York City. No one had thought of using an agency, because promotional models could be supplied from the few who had experience in the field, and at that particular juncture, there were only a handful. Those models were to promote the product as well as model it. The market was expanding so rapidly that there simply weren't enough trained people to fill the need. The entrepreneur started to collect the names and telephone numbers of the women whom she knew had done a little modeling; she contacted some whom she thought would suit the needs of the companies who would hire the models. Due to the demand being by the week or even by the day, the agency had a nice little business going in almost no time at all. The models merely "registered" and then were contacted when this sporadic work arose. There were as many as dozens getting work through this agency daily, where everyone without an inside connection had had to scramble around looking for work through the manufacturers' offices every Monday. It really was a great idea, it benefitted models and the companies who needed these particular models on short notice. The fees are usually a small per cent of your daily income, as almost all of this type of promotional live modeling is paid by the hour. This particular agency is the simplest and least complex of them. The agent was continuing her work as a promotional model and supervising the agency as well. Her specializing in a certain field worked for her because she knew that field very well.

This pattern has occurred repeatedly in people's transitions from modeling into owning agencies or managing models. The model who feels that he or she has a knack for business (and that is strictly what agents are all about) could put to use all the experience from the modeling years.

HOW TO START AN AGENCY

You will probably start with renting or buying some business space. If you plan to have several divisions within the agency, you will need a reasonable amount of space. If you intend to specialize, you can get by with as little as one room with the receptionist, secretary, booker, and you! The bare necessities are the needed equipment. How you attract your clients and models will be your most challenging problem, due to the intense competition.

You have to make certain that your chosen location will have the aura of chic, as that is the product that you are selling. If your office is too far from a high-class neighborhood, neither clients nor models will take you as being adept in your field. Organization is very important, too; you want to keep close track of your models and your clients.

If an agent isn't extremely busy, he or she will be out of business. Working on a percentage can be a pittance unless you represent hundreds of models on that percentage, and then you can be assured of more than a lovely income.

As a model who plans to enter the business world, you have to arm yourself with a completely different way of thinking. You will do well to take a few business courses and scan the general information in the course offerings from business schools. There are also advisory boards whose members are retired business executives. Their wisdom could guide you into the right path without endless trial-and-error.

Financially, you will have to consider the rent, telephone, receptionist, bookkeeper, secretary or two, advertising, cost of furnishings, salaries of employees, taxes, many booking and telephone operators for your models and clients, and general office and business machines. You should visit an agency or two comparable to the type and size of the agency that you are planning. As a current (or past) model, you have a good idea of the inner workings of an agency, but if you've been working as much as most models, there are a lot of details that would have slipped by you. That was what *you* were paying your agent to do, to see to the smooth running of the agency so that you were free to do your end of the work.

Many modeling agencies in the large cities are located near one another. The most chic area of the city usually is where you'll find them. Unfortunately, that means that to move near them, you'll have to pay the highest rents.

The modeling business being what it is guarantees tough competition among modeling agencies for the advertisements. The money to be earned is so stupendous that every agency is vying for a larger and larger slice of the pie. If they weren't aggressive, there wouldn't be any jobs for you or them, and they'd be out looking for other work if they couldn't handle the struggle for power.

It is not really possible to know if you have the type of personality that can cope with all the wheeling and dealing, but it's certainly not a consideration to take lightly unless you are planning to have the one and only agency in an entire area.

HOW TO START A MODELING SCHOOL

Owning a modeling school could be a great deal of fun, accompanied by equal hard work. Depending on its location, a school could need certification from state boards and from local boards. To find out the requirements in your area, write to your state's capital for that information. A modeling school is also considered a business and thus has to pass certain standards according to the Bureau of Consumer Frauds and Protection and the Better Business Bureau.

In New York State "dancing, music, pure or fine art, dramatic art," need not be licensed by the state, according to the New York State Education Law, Section 5001. This ruling pertains to New York only and thus should be a consideration for anyone contemplating the opening of a modeling or charm school in New York state. Other states have different requirements.

You have to judge whether the area where you want to locate will support a school of this nature. In some areas, you might find a mere handful of students, which would

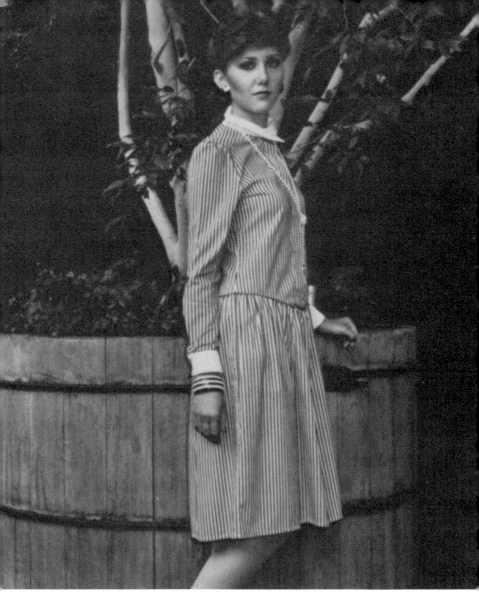

As an agent you might want to specialize in the kinds of models for whom there is plentiful work in your area. Photo: Martha Wodka, Chic, Inc.

necessitate your expanding the school to teaching other curriculum, expanding to include other age groups, or folding.
The possibilities should all be carefully weighed before in-
vesting a penny. Some sections of the country still do not
take any interest in fashion.

After you have tested the waters and found the area to
be fertile to the idea of a charm or modeling school, select
the location and amount of space accordingly. You may
hope to get contracts for advertising from local merchants
after you produce a few polished models who could work
for them. This bit of confirmation might help you decide if
expansion plans could be part of your near future.

What courses will you offer? Can you teach them all
yourself? If this is to be a very small enterprise, then you
probably can do the instruction.

Finances should be a major consideration. It may take
quite a while to get out of the red. Schools can be very successful, but expenses can also be high—rent payment, in-
surance, telephone bill, receptionist, advertising, textbook
(usually one of your own making), electric bill, rental for
video equipment, cameras, makeup, faculty (usually professionals in specialized areas), and allotted amounts for guest
lecturers to keep the instruction up-to-date. Fashion itself is
only that if it is fresh and new.

Publications on fashion around the world also have to be
included in the budget. Imported periodicals are very expensive but are so important in learning where fashion is
established and what each country contributes to the overall
look that is created. Exposure to the fashion world should
include both imported and domestic publications.

Instructing is very different than modeling, of course.
Patience is indispensable, and the desire to help someone
else to learn and understand is the priority. If you feel that
you would enjoy teaching, you could even do some

volunteer work in that area. Though it obviously would not be like giving your own courses, it might provide insight into a field that really is not known for its ease. There have been hundreds of masters in their own select fields who not only realized that they were miscast as instructors in those fields, but truly hated the teaching end of the professions that they adored as performers.

Give serious thought to the possibility of running a school; then if you still feel that you'd like to try running a school but loathe the instruction part, you could hire instructors and enjoy the administration end of things.

WHAT KIND OF MONEY COULD BE MADE FROM OWNING OR MANAGING A MODELING SCHOOL OR AN AGENCY?

The smallest agencies in the tiniest towns make the most insignificant incomes in their chosen fields, due to limited clientele and, often, lack of general interest in fashion. When you look into the possibilities of opening a modeling school or an agency, look through the past few years of the local yellow pages and see how many schools and agencies have not continued to exist in your area. There may be very good reasons *why* the area does not have any modeling establishments. The economy has caused hundreds of these businesses to fold in the past few years. Agencies and schools of modeling that were fairly well established have suddenly disappeared from sight. So thoroughly investigate any area where you think that a modeling business may be just the thing. There is potentially a great deal of money to be earned in the business end of this field. The more clever you are, the better your chances of success.

A modeling agency in a small town could make as little as $10,000 while a modeling school could possibly do the same or better. A medium-sized city would have more people from which to draw both students and clients. For an agency to survive, there have to be both merchants in goodly numbers and models from which the client can choose. The risks are greater, and so are the potential profits.

To give you an idea of how an agency makes its money, consider the following: An average model in a medium-sized city is currently making about $7,000 per year. The agency should have at least a few dozen models capable of this income. The agency collects between ten and fifteen per cent of their job incomes as its fee. Given all the expenses of running the business of the agency, the money could be pretty tight. Certain areas of our country are still doing a large amount of the entire modeling industry. New York City, Los Angeles, Chicago, Dallas, and a handful of the middle-sized cities are the main hubs. These centers seem to be the better business spots for starting an agency or a school of modeling, although you also encounter greater competition from other existing schools and agencies by locating there.

Several famous models have opened their own agencies in these largest of cities and are doing very well. In fact, many of the most well-known modeling agencies in New York City are owned and run by former models. They are very successful businesswomen and extremely adept managers. Super-models are rare, but super-modeling agents and their agencies are even more rare. But you may *be* that one in millions who has the shrewdness and business sense to start and keep a large agency afloat.

There are also smaller agencies, specialist agencies, and even an agency run as a franchise. You might want to consider these possibilities too.

The most popular franchises are the modeling schools, and the income there would depend greatly on your ability to attract students. There would obviously be better locations than others. These schools are scattered over the 50 states, as required by the population centers. The lowest-paying ownerships or franchises would run around $15,000 per annum, and the largest incomes in owning your own modeling agency would be well up in the millions.

Owning a modeling agency is not everybody's forte. The stress is incredible, and the competition deadly. You may want to look into other possible related work than owning or managing a modeling facility, but you are your own best judge. There are very successful agents out there. You may have it in you to be one also!

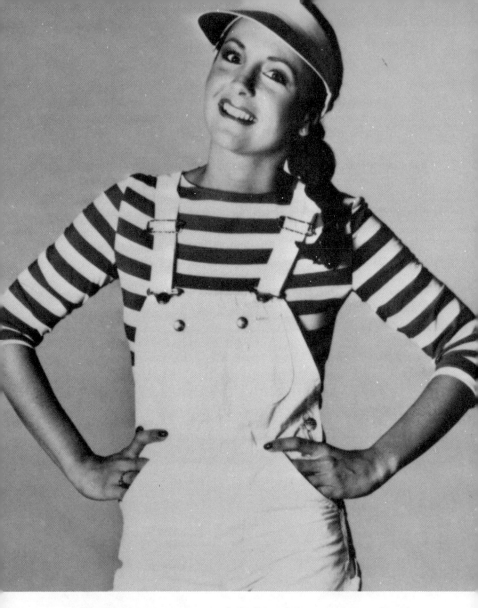

Active, athletic poses have been emphasized recently in more and more print and television advertising. Photo: Lesley Schwartz, Chic, Inc.

CHAPTER 10

THE FUTURE OF MODELING

As long as the United States remains a product-oriented society the necessity for models will prevail. People use products, and the picture being worth a thousand words has paid off handsomely for manufacturers. From toothpaste to Rolls Royces, from diapers to diamonds, we are accustomed to seeing an attractive person positioned with the salable item as a supposedly believable consumer.

The amount of work for models in all categories is on the rise. There were 50,000 working models in the United States in 1979. That number rose to 60,000 working models who were totally dependent on their incomes as professionals in 1980! The New York State Department of Labor, who supplied these figures, says that most of these models are located in and around New York City and "other large cities."

Promotional modeling alone has taken a giant step forward in the past few years. This particular area has created thousands of new jobs. The field encompasses models in department stores, trade shows, and even television.

MALE MODELS IN GREAT DEMAND

Male modeling also expanded tremendously in the 1980s. The major modeling agencies have all opened divisions for their male models due to the expanded new market. Men are now working as runway models for shows and videos, doing print and live work, and edging into the fashion world that had been dominated exclusively by the female models for decades.

The emergence of the male as an admired figure for his looks alone is a new trend, and the male modeling world is capitalizing on this idea. The male model no longer needs to be a gentleman shown in a size 40 suit, as an accessory to an exquisitely turned out high fashion female model, but is more often seen as an entity unto himself. He has the whole gamut of a designer-made wardrobe. Underwear for men has become very status-oriented, and as a result many male models are being hired for their beautiful physiques. This was not the case just a few years ago, when the male model's major purpose was to render a subdued but proper costume, an inspired necessity to any man's wardrobe.

The recent trend toward fashion design in men's apparel has led major newspapers to do extensive sections on menswear from hats to swimwear.

The look that is currently all the rage is the clean-cut boy-next-door, collegiate-athlete. Very short, slicked down hair is reminiscent of the 1930s, though with a more relaxed overall attitude. The wardrobe of the modern male has expanded to such incredible dimensions that men's cosmetics, fragrances, and facial products are an immense market in themselves. Both the live and photographic male models are needed for this ballooning market.

Color is another major change in the men's clothing market. It is not unusual to have the wardrobe include every color of shirt, pants, ties, and jackets that could be imagined. Therefore, the prints and catalogs are now much more extensive than they used to be and are creating more and more work for the male model. The variety of sports-

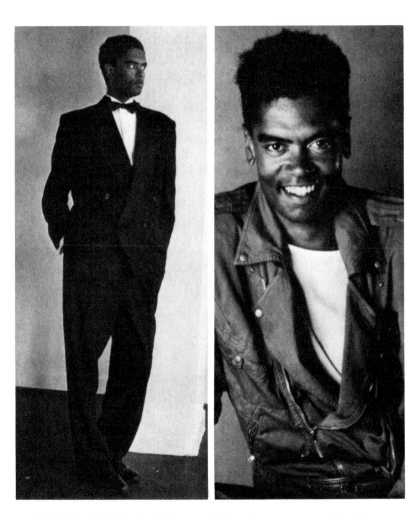

Model Chazz is six feet, four inches; can do formal or sportswear equally well.
Photo: Star Model Management; photographers, left, Ben Sederowsky, and right,
Tom Lee.

wear alone fills pages of ads in magazines, catalogs, newspapers, and on billboards and flyers.

Men's shoes, boots, and sports footwear have become so diversified that they are now classified as fashion also and get lots of prime ad space.

Eyewear has become so chic that men are expected to sport several different kinds of sunglasses, as well as designer frames if they do not wear contact lenses.

The high-priced men's clothing market has created thousands of modeling spots. The items are so status-oriented that many are one-of-a-kind. Much male modeling has become prestigious in the same way that female modeling has. Items that were exclusively worn by the super-rich of yesterday are a fast growing market for today's man. Silk pajamas, linen shorts, elegant shawl-collared robes that sell for hundreds are fast becoming chic for men.

The well-dressed man of yesterday was more than likely quietly outfitted by his tailor exclusively, and there was no need to advertise style as it was set by the famous and royal. Today's man is able to dress with much more flair than ever before, and the selection is shown endlessly by the male modeling industry.

It would not be unusual for a male model to make well over $50,000 per year after he started to become established. If he "takes off," his salary could well be over the $100,000 mark. There are men who model the gamut from photographic work to television commercials. They do extremely well at paycheck time and are able to maintain their careers for many years.

Male models are needed very frequently for catalog work. This can be their bread-and-butter for decades if they are liked by the client and remain attractive. Men's clothing, unlike women's, does not change style dramatically each year.

Modeling schools accept male models-to-be at age thirteen and upward. This would not be an option in all schools, as some instruct only women. Many schools feel that the male model is mostly interested in television commercials and thus stress that particular area of instruction for men. The television commercial is one of the highest paying areas for the male model, without doubt. The other area where he might stand to make a large amount for one commercial would be in the contract for an exclusive product (similar to that of the Marlboro Man). These are the two that stand alone at the top of the ladder.

A male model could be hired by an agency at anywhere from about $175 to $300 per hour as his starting rate. If he becomes popular, his rate increases. An agency will help polish a man into a model if they feel that he has the potential; it will also help with portfolio guidance and with his photographs, making appointments with photographers who may be testing.

The male model today is a whole different professional than just five years ago. We are in the midst of a fashion revolution for men. Men are suddenly wearing the brightest or at least comparable colors; leathers are worn as slacks, shirts, and even hats. There are men involved in every area of the fashion industry, and they're no longer making all those fancy items for just women. The modeling industry now parallels what is being created in the men's fashion world. And as a result, both are really booming!

THE FUTURE OF MODELING FOR WOMEN MODELS

Women models have always had the corner on the market, and they are still increasing in numbers in all categories. Women models tend to take advantage of their ability to work in the various markets throughout the world. They also go back and forth when other work, like a television role, is offered. While increases are shown in the number of female models registered, the actual employment of female models has not grown much on an annual basis.

Many women models are branching out into the entire spectrum of modeling possibilities to make as much money as is available while they are employable in the field.

The newest market for the female model is that of video, which is an ever increasing market. The high fashion model is getting much more exposure via the video than ever before.

The other area that has opened up expressly for the female model is the area of high fashion with extremely young women showing women's couture (fashion). These young girls are taking over a market that had been solely reserved for women at least ten years older. It has placed a whole different vantage point on the modeling future. If young women of ages 11 to 13 are to be the representatives of the high fashion market, the prices that they command will fall in the highest ranges. There are contracts offered and signed now that are in the hundreds of thousands for the right look in the preteen years. This trend started about seven years ago and has taken off. Now all the major agencies are hiring younger and younger girls who would normally be employed by an agency for children's modeling.

Salary rates per hour doubled in many instances between 1979 and 1983. Catalog work was paying $75 per hour versus today's pay scale of $150. Children now make $75 per hour for catalog work. Many models are now started at pay scales of $300 per hour, and the scale rises with demand for the model!

Women models have more choices today than they have

ever had. The increase in salary per hour has been a big step forward, but the opportunity to work in hundreds of different locations has also expanded the viable market. Many young women who would have been limited to working in New York City are working in many major cities in Europe, Scandinavia, Australia, Japan, and other large cities in the United States.

The market is larger, the work is more varied, and regardless of the immense numbers of men and children who are joining the modeling force, modeling is still the stronghold of a woman's industry. There are many more job opportunities in the modeling field for young women than for any of the other members of the profession. Pretty young women will be in demand to promote the nation's products, as long as the American industrial world and a large portion of the advertising industry believe that sexy young women attract both men and women to products.

THE FUTURE OF TELEVISION MODELING

Television modeling is another area that is burgeoning beyond all predictions for making money as a model. There are more possibilities for variety in this medium than any of the others. The man who is a he-man, wimp, pizza-tosser, or skydiver can make large amounts from television commercials.

For the women models, anything from high fashion to the hands-only are possible. All areas for women are soaring. There is no shortage of work in television, but there is endless competition. Everybody wants a slice of the most well-paying pie.

Male models are making a much more obvious stand in television commercials, as their clothing goes more and more into designer fashions. The men's cosmetic industry is taking off, as is the entire array of leisure items from home computers to sporting gear.

Child models are also doing extremely well, from tiny babies to teenagers. Their field encompasses the major portion of the toy market (which is sizable), children's clothing and shoes, medicines for children, and a myriad of other possibilities. In fact the market is so lucrative that many child models are surpassing their counterparts in the adult modeling world. *Everyone loves puppies and babies* is an old adage, but it has paid its weight in gold in the television commercial world. Recently a baby only a few months old made over $13,000 in commercials and their residuals.

The area of television commercials has so expanded that many major modeling agencies that handled basically photographic models have now added separate television divisions to their ranks. Many models used to have the modeling agency do the booking for everything except television commercials and now are able to have their modeling agent handle the whole market. Agents and managers who do not run modeling agencies also handle television commercial people.

Television has a very solid future and promises many jobs for models of both sexes and the widest variety of ages. The television industry runs on the money of sponsors, and they are in continual need of models to demonstrate their products.

Models and actors used to be looked down upon for doing commercials, but the money and attitudes have both changed noticeably. The biggest names in show business are out there as your stiffest competition for that high-paying commercial.

The money gleaned from television commercials totalled around $350 million in 1982. It has been estimated that producers of items used to clean and keep up your house spent over $60,000 billion in their advertisements on television in 1982. The future of the television commercial business is very good and looking better annually.

APPENDIX A

MODELING SCHOOLS AND AGENCIES

In the following pages you will find a listing of some of the modeling agents and schools. If you happen to live in, or plan to visit, an area where one of them is located, write ahead and ask what procedure they follow. Many places do not like photographs sent and prefer a live interview. Many prefer exactly the opposite, in that they want to see photographs first. They may then contact you for more or better prints, and *then* may want to set up an appointment to see you. So as not to waste your time or the time of the agency, do make initial contact by letter or by phone. Never just drop in. Hundreds of young hopefuls are waiting to get into modeling agencies. The staff is usually very polite and helpful; so contact them, let them know what you'd like to accomplish with their agency's help and let them advise you.

Many contacts are made months ahead so that all the preparations will be completed by the time that they are needed. If you are planning a vacation to a large city, and you want to set up interviews, you'll be ahead of the game if you come equipped with a face-on head shot, 3/4 head shot, full length shot or whatever is requested. Thinking ahead could put you at the agency at the opportune moment. Much depends on timing. Do not feel, even if you are accepted by the agency, that you are under pressure to sign instantly. Several young models-to-be have been signed and then have started to work full-time as soon as another obligation—school, job, or whatever—was completed. If the agency wants you, be honest about what you want from them, and when.

A PARTIAL LIST OR SAMPLING OF AREA SCHOOLS AND AGENCIES IN THE UNITED STATES

An *S* after name indicates *school;* and an *A* indicates *agency.*

ALABAMA

Birmingham

Alabama School of Modeling(S)
210 S. 18th St.
Birmingham, AL 35233

ALASKA

Anchorage

John Robert Powers(S)
750 West 2nd St.
Anchorage, AK 99501

ARIZONA

Phoenix

L'Image Agency(A)
7220 Stetson Dr.
Scottsdale, AZ 85251

Plaza Three Modeling & Finishing(S,A)
School & Talent & Modeling Agency
4343 N. 16th St.
Phoenix, AZ 85016

CALIFORNIA

Beverly Hills

Flaire Agency(S,A)
8693 Wilshire Blvd.
Beverly Hills, CA 90212

Hollywood

Caroline Leonetti Ltd.(A,S)
6526 W. Sunset Blvd.
Hollywood, CA 90028

Los Angeles

CHN International Agency(A)
7428 Santa Monica Blvd.
Los Angeles, CA 90046

California Girls
1855 Lincoln Blvd.
Santa Monica, CA 90045

John Robert Powers(S)
1533 Wilshire Blvd.
Los Angeles, CA 90017

Nina Blanchard Agency(A)
1717 N. Highland Ave.
Los Angeles, CA 90028

Show Talent International
  Agency(A)
Artist's Manager
831 Fairfax Ave.
Los Angeles, CA 90046

San Diego

John Casablancas Model
  Center(A)
409 Camino Real Del Rio S.
San Diego, CA 92108

John Robert Powers School(A)
2225 Camino Del Rio S.
San Diego, CA 92108

Tina Real Talent Agency(A)
3108 Fifth Ave.
San Diego, CA 92103

San Francisco

Barbizon School of Modeling
  & Fashion Merchandising(S)
447 Sutter
San Francisco, CA 94108

Bianca Modeling(A)
260 Stockton
San Francisco, CA 94108

Grimme School of Fashion
  Modeling
214 Grant Ave.
San Francisco, CA 94108

John Casablancas Elite Center
536 Sutter
San Francisco, CA 94108

COLORADO

Denver

Image Improvement
10673 E. Powers Dr.
Denver, CO 80232

J.F. Images Inc.(S,A)
3600 S. Yosemite
Denver, CO 80237

Fort Collins

Elan School of Modeling(S)
333 W. Drake
Fort Collins, CO 80221

CONNECTICUT

Stamford

Connecticut Modeling
  Agency(A)
1326 Shippan Ave.
Stamford, CN 06902

FLORIDA

Fort Lauderdale

Act I Casting Agency(A)
1460 Brickel Ave.
Fort Lauderdale, FL 33301

Barbizon School of
  Modeling(S)
950 N.E. 62nd St.
Fort Lauderdale, FL 33304

Florida Talent Agency(A)
2631 E. Oakland Pk. Blvd.
Fort Lauderdale, FL 33306

Marbea Talent(A)
104 Crandon Blvd.
Key Biscayne, FL 33304

A Central Casting of
  Florida(A)
411 N.E. 11th Ave.
Fort Lauderdale, FL 33304

Miami

Fashioncrest
  International(A,S)
777 N.W. 72nd Ave.
Miami, FL 33126

Glyne Kennedy Talent(A)
1828 N.E. 4th Ave.
Miami, FL 33138

Miami Beach

Falcon Travis Modeling
  Agency(A)
17070 Collins Ave.
Miami Beach, FL 33160

Tampa

Barbizon of Tampa
219 Mariner Sq.
Tampa, FL 33609

Carol Berg Ultimate Talent(A)
8313 W. Hillsborough
Tampa, FL 33615

Evelyn Stewarts' Florida Model
  Center & Agency(A)
9361 N. Florida Ave.
Tampa, FL 33612

Model's Ltd.(A)
5610 Hanley Rd.
Tampa, FL 33614

New Image Center
3918 E. Hillsborough
Tampa, FL 33610

GEORGIA

Atlanta

Austons Professional Modeling
  of Atlanta Inc.
550 Pharr Rd. N.E.
Atlanta, GA 30305

HAWAII

Honolulu

Barbizon of Hawaii(S)
1600 Kapiolani Blvd.
Honolulu, HI 16821

ILLINOIS

Champaign

Johnson & Johnson Beauty
  Unlimited(A)
201 E. Sangamon Rantoul
Champaign, IL 61820

Chicago

Barbizon of Chicago(S)
303 E. Ohio
Chicago, IL 60611

Chic Inc.(A)
1207 N. State St.
Chicago, IL 60610

David Lee Models(A)
64 E. Walton
Chicago, IL 60611

The Geddes Agency(A)
1522 Hancock Center
Chicago, IL 60611

Shirley Hamilton Inc.(A)
620 N. Michigan
Chicago, IL 60611

Hospitality Services, Inc.(A)
1030 N. State
Chicago, IL 60611

John Robert Powers(S)
27 E. Monroe
Chicago, IL 60603

Playboy Model Agency(A)
919 N. Michigan Ave.
Chicago, IL 60611

Stewart Talent Agency(A)
70 W. Hubbard
Chicago, IL 60611

INDIANA

Evansville

CST Fashion Academy(S)
Old Court House
Evansville, IN 47708

Indianapolis

The Agency(A)
3843 N. Meridian
Indianapolis, IN 46208

John Robert Powers(S)
7 N. Meridian St.
Indianapolis, IN 46204

IOWA

Des Moines

All Iowa Model Guide(S)
3711 Blane
Des Moines, IA 50310

Curtis Studios
1168½ 24th St.
Des Moines, IA 50311

MARYLAND

Baltimore

Barbizon School of
Modeling(S)
One Investment Pl.
Towson, MD 21204

Patricia Stevens Institute of
Fashion(S)
Eastpoint Mall
Baltimore, MD 21228

Patricia Stevens Institute of
Fashions(S)
Westview Mall
Baltimore, MD 21228

Plaza Modeling & Talent
  Agency(A)
400 Virginia Ave.
Baltimore, MD 21204

MASSACHUSETTS
Boston
Agency for Models(A)
108A Appleton
Boston, MA 02116

American Residuals & Talent
  Inc.(A)
69 Newbury St.
Boston, MA 02116

Barbizon Schools of Modeling
  & Fashion(S)
739 Boylston St.
Boston, MA 02116

Cameo Modeling & Talent
  Agency(A)
392 Boylston St.
Boston, MA 02116

Carol Nashe(A)
228 Beacon
Boston, MA 02116

Hart Agency Inc.(A)
137 Newbury
Boston, MA 02116

John Robert Powers Model
  Management
304 Boylston St.
Boston, MA 02116

Models Consultant
163 Marlboro
Boston, MA 02116

Weymouth

Carole McColes Fashion
  Models School & Agency
572 Columbian
Weymouth, MA 02190

MICHIGAN
Detroit
London Studio(A)
10095 Gratiot
Detroit, MI 48213

Plymouth
Detroit Modeling Agency(A)
496 W. Ann Arbor Tri.
Plymouth, MI 48170

Troy
Patricia Stevens
  Casting Agency(A)
1900 W. Big Beaver
Troy, MI 48084

NEW YORK
Buffalo
Barbizon School of Modeling,
  Inc.(A,S)
740 Statler Building
Buffalo, NY 14202

June II Model Agency(A)
143½ Allen St.
Buffalo, NY 14202

New York City
Barbizon Agency(S,A)
3 E. 54th St.
New York, NY 10022

Big Beauties(A)
159 Madison Ave.
New York, NY 10028

Bonnie Kid Models(A)
250 W. 57th St.
New York, NY 10019

Click Model Agency(A)
881 Seventh Ave.
New York, NY

Ophelia DeVore School of
Charm(S)
1697 Broadway
New York, NY 10019

Elite Model Management
Corp.(A)
150 E. 58th St.
New York, NY 10022

Elite Men's Division(A)
150 E. 58th St.
New York, NY 10022

Ford Men(A)
344 E. 59th St.
New York, NY 10022

Ford Models, Inc.(A)
344 E. 59th St.
New York, NY 10022

Foster-Fell Inc.(A)
26 W. 38th St.
New York, NY 10018

Funny Face(A)
527 Madison Ave.
New York, NY 10022

Anthony Greene Model
Management(A)
245 E. 63rd St.
New York, NY 10021

Ellen Harth, Inc.(A)
149 Madison Ave.
New York, NY 10022

International Model Agency(A)
232 Madison Ave.
New York, NY 10016

International Top Model
Agency(A)
677 Fifth Ave.
New York, NY 10022

L'Agence(A)
12 W. 57th St.
New York, NY 10019

Mannequin Models Inc.(A)
730 Fifth Ave.
New York, NY 10019

Marge McDermott Enterprises
Agency(A)
216 E. 39th St.
New York, NY 10016

Models Service Agency(A)
1457 Broadway
New York, NY 10036

Perkins Models(A)
1697 Broadway
New York, NY 10010

Plus Model Management(A)
49 W. 37th St.
New York, NY 10018

John Robert Powers School(S)
119 W. 57th St.
New York, NY 10019

Wally Rogers(A)
160 E. 56th St.
New York, NY 10022

Gilla Roos(A)
527 Madison Ave.
New York, NY 10022

Charles V. Ryan Enterprises(A)
200 W. 57th St.
New York, NY 10019

William Schuller Agency,
Inc.(A)
667 Madison Ave.
New York, NY 10021

Smith School of Modeling(S)
171 Madison Ave.
New York, NY 10016

Summa Models(A)
250 W. 57th St.
New York, NY 10019

Van Der Veer Models(A)
225 A East 59th St.
New York, NY 10022

Wilhelmina Models Inc.(A)
9 E. 37th St.
New York, NY 10016

Ann Wright Representatives(A)
136 E. 57th St.
New York, NY 10022

Zoli Models Inc.(A)
146 E. 56th St.
New York, NY 10021

NORTH CAROLINA

Asheboro

Papillon School of Modeling(S)
P.O. Box 1505
208 Sunset Ave.
Asheboro, NC 27203

OHIO

Cleveland

Artha-Jon Academy of
Modeling & Charm(S)
2800 Euclid Ave.
Cleveland, OH 44115

Barbizon School of Cleveland
Inc.(S,A)
110 Terminal Tower
Cleveland, OH 44113

Cleveland's Cream Inc.(A)
14809 Kinsman
Cleveland, OH 44120

David Lee Modeling Agency(A)
1801 E. 12th St.
Cleveland, OH 44114

Gary Von Agency(A)
25700 Lorain Rd.
Cleveland, OH 44113

John Robert Powers School &
Agency(A,S)
1290 Euclid Ave.
Cleveland, OH 44115

Professional Modeling
  Service(A)
29525 Chagrin Blvd.
Cleveland, OH 44122

Sid Fried Man's Modeling
  Agency(A)
Statler Office Towers
Cleveland, OH 44101

Columbus

Barbizon Modeling
  Agency(A,S)
370 South 5th St.
Columbus, OH 43215

Kathleen Busche
School/Prestige Agency(A,S)
1720 East Broad St.
Columbus, OH 43203

Jeanette Grider School of
  Modeling(S)
1453 East Main St.
Columbus, OH 43205

Noni Agency(A)
209 South High St.
Columbus, OH 43215

John Robert Powers School &
  Agency(S,A)
5900 Roche Dr., Suite 205
Columbus, OH 43229

Wright Models(A,S)
4100 North High St.
Columbus, OH 43214

Dayton

Bette Massie Inc.(A)
261 North Main St.
Dayton, OH 45402

Glamour School &
  Agency(A,S)
140 North Main St.
Dayton, OH 45402

Sharkey Agency Inc.(A,S)
1299 Lyons Rd.
Dayton, OH 45402

PENNSYLVANIA

Philadelphia

Barbizon School of
  Modeling(A,S)
1520 Walnut St.
Philadelphia, PA 19102

John Barth Casting(A)
Broad and Locust
Philadelphia, PA 19101

John Robert Powers(S)
1425 Chestnut St.
Philadelphia, PA 19103

Ruth Harper's Modeling and
  Charm School(S,A)
1427 West Erie Ave.
Philadelphia, PA 19107

Kay Models
1647 Harrison
Philadelphia, PA 19102

Pittsburgh

A Models Unlimited
1701 Banksville Rd.
Pittsburgh, PA 15216

AAA Van Enterprises
Fulton Bldg.
Pittsburgh, PA 15222

Entertainment Unlimited
1701 Banksville Rd.
Pittsburgh, PA 15216

Pittsburgh Pennsylvania Model
  Directory
100 Brownsville
Pittsburgh, PA 15238

The Wheeler School
212 9th St.
Pittsburgh, PA 15222

RHODE ISLAND

Providence

Barbizon Models
169 Weybst
Providence, RI 02903

Bella Advertising and Fashions
  Inc.
530 Industrial Bank Bldg.
Providence, RI 02903

SOUTH CAROLINA

Columbia

Buffette Models Workshop
4021 Monticello
Columbia, SC 29203

Collins Models-Studio &
  Agency
1441 Greenhill Rd.
Columbia, SC 29206

Millie Lewis Modeling
Finishing School &
  Agency(A,S)
3022 Milwood Ave.
Columbia, SC 29205

Greenville

Millie Lewis Modeling Agency
Diran Executive Plaza
850 S. Pleasantburg Dr.
Greenville, SC 29607

TENNESSEE

Chattanooga

Chaparral Talent Agency
P.O. Box 25
Chattanooga, TN 37363

Studio V
523 Lupton Dr.
Chattanooga, TN 37415

Germantown

Barbizon School of
  Modeling(A,S)
Kirby Woods Mall
Germantown, TN 38138

Memphis

Dot's Modeling Studios &
  Agency
1880 Lamar Ave.
Memphis, TN 38114

Elite Artists Inc.
3385 Airways Blvd.
Memphis, TN 38116

Patricia Stevens Finishing &
Modeling Career School(S)
1853 Madison Ave.
Memphis, TN 38104

TEXAS

Austin

Adams Studio
7524 N. Lamar
Austin, TX 78752

Angel's Modeling Agency
3705 Vineland Dr.
Austin, TX 78722

Hall Agency
503 W. 15th
Austin, TX 78701

Dallas

Barbizon School of
Modeling(S,A)
12700 Hillcrest
Dallas, TX 75230

Tanya Blair Agency(A)
3000 Carlisle St., Suite 101
Dallas, TX 75202

Celebrity Talent Agency-Artist
Management
1901 Royal Ln.
Dallas, TX 75229

Continental Modeling
Agency(A)
8150 N. Central Expwy.
Dallas, TX 75225

Darry Modeling(S)
6014 Velasco
Dallas, TX 75206

Kim Dawson Agency Artists
Manager(A)
Apparel Mart
Dallas, TX 75207

Joan Frank Models(A)
9950 Forest Ln.
Dallas, TX 75234

Tokyo Modeling Studio
4030 Cedar Springs
Dallas, TX 75219

Peggy Taylor Talent, Inc.(A)
6309 N. O'Connor
Dallas, TX 75206

Sandy's Modeling Studio
1210 Oak Lawn
Dallas, TX 75207

El Paso

Fran Simon Talent & Modeling
9611 Acer
El Paso, TX 79925

Le Fleur Elegant
10600 Gala Pl.
El Paso, TX 79924

Houston

Act I Models
5322 W. Bellfort
Houston, TX 77033

Ashley Film Productions Inc.
730 N. Post Oak Rd.
Houston, TX 77024

Golden Girl Studio
321 W. Alabama
Houston, TX 77006

Sunset Productions
730 N. Post Oak Rd.
Houston, TX 77024

WASHINGTON

Seattle

John Robert Powers(A,S)
1610 Sixth Ave.
Seattle, WA 98101

Kathleen Peck Finishing &
Modeling School/Model
   Agency(A,S)
10843 N.E. 8th
Bellevue, WA 98004

Seattle Models Guild
1610 Sixth
Seattle, WA 98101

Thompson's Models(S,A)
11522 24th St. N.E.
Seattle, WA 98125

WASHINGTON DC

Anne Schwab's Model Store
3122 M St. N.W.
Washington DC 20007

Cappa Chell School &
   Modeling Agency(A,S)
1120 Connecticut Ave. N.W.
Washington DC 20036

TELEVISION COMMERCIAL AGENTS

NEW YORK CITY

Agency for the Performing
  Arts, Inc.
888 7th Ave.
New York, NY 10022

Ann Wright
137 E. 57th St.
New York, NY 10022

Beverly Anderson
1472 Broadway
New York, NY 10036

D.M.I. Talent Associates Ltd.
250 W. 57th St.
New York, NY 10019

Elite Model Management
  Corp.
150 E. 58th St.
New York, NY 10022

Ford Models Inc.
344 E. 59th St.
New York, NY 10022

International Creative
  Management
40 W. 57th St.
New York, NY 10019

Jeff Hunter
119 W. 57th St.
New York, NY 10019

Raglyn Shamsky Talent
  Representatives Ltd.
60 E. 42nd St.
New York, NY 10017

William D. Cunningham &
  Associates, Inc.
919 Third Ave.
New York, NY 10022

William Morris Agency, Inc.
1350 Sixth Ave.
New York, NY 10019

Wilhelmina Models Inc.
9 E. 37th St.
New York, NY 10016

LOS ANGELES

Nina Blanchard Agency
1717 N. Highland Ave.
Los Angeles, CA 90028

J. Michael Bloom
9220 Sunset Blvd.
Los Angeles, CA 90069

William D. Cunningham &
  Associates
216 S. Robertson Blvd.
Beverly Hills, CA 90211

Judith Fontaine Agency
6565 Sunset Blvd.
Hollywood, CA 90028

International Creative
  Management
8899 Beverly
Los Angeles, CA 90048

William Morris
151 El Camino Dr.
Beverly Hills, CA 90212

PUBLICATIONS FOR MODELS

AMERICAN PERIODICALS

Glamour Magazine
350 Madison Ave.
New York, NY 10002

Harpers Bazaar
1700 Broadway
New York, NY 10019

Ladies Home Journal
3 Park Avenue
New York, NY 10016

Seventeen Magazine
850 Third Ave.
New York, NY 10022

Teen Magazine
437 Madison Ave.
New York, NY 10002

Vogue Magazine
350 Madison Ave.
New York, NY 10002

FOREIGN PERIODICALS

Elle
E.D.I., 7 (F.E.P. Hachette et
  Cie.) S.N.C.
  Locataire-gerant
6 Rue Ancelle
92525 Neuilly-Sur-Seine,
  France

Follow me
61-63 Glenmore Rd.
Paddington, 2021. Australia

Marie Claire
11 Bis, Rue Boissy-d'Anglais
75008 Paris, France

Marie Claire Bis
11 Bis, Rue Boissy-d'Anglais
75008 Paris, France

NEWSPAPERS TO THE TRADE

Back Stage
Back Stage Publications
330 W. 42nd St.
New York, NY 10036

Back Stage Midwest
841 N. Addison Ave.
Elmhurst, IL 60126

Back Stage West
5150 Wilshire Blvd.
Los Angeles, CA 90036

Daily Variety
1400 N. Cahuenga Blvd.
Hollywood, CA 90028

Show Business News
136 W. 44th St.
New York, NY 10036

Variety Inc.
154 W. 46th St.
New York, NY 10036

Womens Wear Daily
7 E. 12th St.
New York, NY 10011

APPENDIX D

BIBLIOGRAPHY OF RELATED READING

Griffing, Marie Fenton. *How To Be a Beauty Pageant Winner*. New York: Simon and Schuster, 1981.

Krem, Viju. *How To Become a Successful Model*. New York: ARCO, 1980.

MacGil, Gillis. *Your Future as a Model*. New York: Richard Rosen Press Inc., 1978.

Marlowe, Francine. *Male Modeling: an Inside Look*. Copyright New York: by Barbizon International, Inc. Crown Publishers Inc., 1980.

Stafford, Marilyn. *The Inside Secret to a Modeling Career*. Mid-Coast Publications, 1982.

Walker, Greta. *Modeling Careers: A Concise Career Guide*. New York: Franklin Watts, 1976.

VGM CAREER BOOKS

OPPORTUNITIES IN

Available in both paperback and hardbound editions

Accounting Careers
Acting Careers
Advertising Careers
Airline Careers
Animal and Pet Care
Appraising Valuation Science
Architecture
Automotive Service
Banking
Beauty Culture
Biological Sciences
Book Publishing
Broadcasting Careers
Building Construction Trades
Business Management
C.A.D./C.A.M. Careers
Cable Television
Carpentry
Chemical Engineering
Chemistry
Chiropractic Health Care
Civil Engineering
Commercial Art and Graphic Design
Computer Science Careers
Counseling & Development
Dance
Data Processing Careers
Dental Care
Drafting Careers
Electrical Trades
Electronic and Electrical Engineering
Energy Careers
Engineering Technology
Environmental Careers
Fashion
Federal Government Careers
Film Careers
Financial Careers
Fire Protection Services
Fitness Careers
Food Services
Foreign Language Careers
Forestry Careers

Free Lance Writing
Government Service
Graphic Communications
Health and Medical Careers
Hospital Administration
Hotel & Motel Management
Industrial Design
Interior Design
Journalism Careers
Landscape Architecture
Law Careers
Law Enforcement and Criminal Justice
Library and Information Science
Machine Shop Trades
Magazine Publishing
Management
Marine & Maritime
Materials Science
Mechanical Engineering
Microelectronics
Modeling Careers
Music Careers
Nursing Careers
Nutrition Careers
Occupational Therapy
Office Occupations
Opticianry
Optometry
Packaging Science
Paralegal Careers
Paramedical Careers
Personnel Management
Pharmacy Careers
Photography
Physical Therapy
Podiatric Medicine
Printing Careers
Psychiatry
Psychology
Public Relations Careers
Real Estate
Recreation and Leisure
Refrigeration and Air Conditioning
Religious Service
Sales & Marketing
Secretarial Careers

Securities Industry
Sports & Athletics
Sports Medicine
State and Local Government
Teaching Careers
Technical Communications
Telecommunications
Theatrical Design & Production
Transportation
Travel Careers
Veterinary Medicine
Word Processing
Writing Careers
Your Own Service Business

WOMEN IN

Available in both paperback and hardbound editions

Communications
Engineering
Finance
Government
Management
Science
Their Own Business

CAREER PLANNING

How to Get People to Do Things Your Way
How to Land a Better Job
How to Write a Winning Résumé
Life Plan
Planning Your Career of Tomorrow
Planning Your College Education
Planning Your Military Career
Planning Your Own Home Business
Planning Your Young Child's Education

SURVIVAL GUIDES

High School Survival Guide
College Survival Guide

 VGM Career Horizons
A Division of National Textbook Company
4255 West Touhy Avenue
Lincolnwood, Illinois 60646-1975 U.S.A.